SHAMANIC HEALING

"This intriguing book is a call to action and a challenge to integrate shamanic knowledge about health care with modern science. Itzhak's latest contribution to this body of wisdom guides us along that path. I highly recommend it."

JOHN PERKINS, AUTHOR OF THE NEW YORK TIMES BESTSELLER
CONFESSIONS OF AN ECONOMIC HIT MAN

"*Shamanic Healing* is an important book for the times we live in, as so many people in the Western world are searching for alternative ways of healing. This book provides a wealth of shamanic healing methods from indigenous cultures that can be integrated into anyone's life and/or their work with clients. Itzhak Beery did a brilliant job bringing this work to us."

SANDRA INGERMAN, M.A., AUTHOR OF SOUL RETRIEVAL
AND SPEAKING WITH NATURE

"Belief structures tend to put a fence around our consciousness, as Itzhak Beery shows in his new book on shamanic healing. He creates a bridge between ideals that no longer serve us and the ancient, yet current, practices of ancient shamanism up until today. Beery's book offers a new model to transform our sick care into holistic health care."

LYNN V. ANDREWS, AUTHOR OF COMING FULL CIRCLE

"In *Shamanic Healing,* Itzhak Beery has created an extraordinary book that records generous teachings brought to life through his accounts of adventures and healing stories from which readers may extract techniques and insights that may enrich their lives. Itzhak is a medicine man, and he has created very good medicine indeed. "

HANK WESSELMAN, PH.D., ANTHROPOLOGIST,
AUTHOR OF THE SPIRITWALKER TRILOGY,
AND COAUTHOR OF AWAKENING TO THE SPIRIT WORLD

"*Shamanic Healing* supports the ongoing revolution in health, as the modern world discovers alternative methods can be effective for many types of maladies—physical, psychological, and even spiritual. Itzhak Beery's book provides a clear, coherent introduction and overview of these ancient practices, which are evermore popular."

DANIEL PINCHBECK, AUTHOR OF *HOW SOON IS NOW?*

"Through crisp narrative and excellent storytelling, Itzhak Beery takes on the timely and powerful subject of shamanic healing and its relevance in our modern world. In a world where we find our medical model bankrupt and too often causing illness and death instead of healing, people are seeking alternatives, including the ancient, effective ways of shamanism. Here you will find an excellent and comprehensive introduction to the world of shamanic healing based on South American traditions. His book is a real contribution to shamanic literature."

JOSÉ LUIS STEVENS, PH.D.,
AUTHOR OF *ENCOUNTERS WITH POWER*

"Izhak Beery's passionate love of shamanism gives us a glimpse at how rich and fulfilling shamanic work can be in one's life. He writes with an urgency to embed shamanic healing practices into our Western world, so we may align all our senses harmoniously with the supportive energies of the Earth and assure the survival of our species. An excellent book for all who seek to deepen their understanding of shamanic healing practices."

TOM COWAN, AUTHOR OF *FIRE IN THE HEAD*

"Itzhak Beery has written a spectacular book. This honest, nonlinear journey into the very heart and soul of shamanism rekindled my heart's flame and strengthened my commitment to the shamanic path that we share."

LINDA STAR WOLF, PH.D., COAUTHOR OF *SOUL WHISPERING*

"Itzhak Beery's heart and compassion encompass all of his teachings, and his fierce commitment to the integrity of this work is an inspiration to all who come in contact with him. His brilliant writing will open you to the beauty and elegance of walking the shamanic path."

MICHAEL STONE, TEACHER, ACTIVIST,
WRITER, AND RADIO HOST

SHAMANIC HEALING

Traditional Medicine *for the* Modern World

ITZHAK BEERY

Destiny Books
Rochester, Vermont • Toronto, Canada

Destiny Books
One Park Street
Rochester, Vermont 05767
www.DestinyBooks.com

Destiny Books is a division of Inner Traditions International

Copyright © 2017 by Itzhak Beery

All rights reserved. No part of this book may be reproduced or utilized in
any form or by any means, electronic or mechanical, including photocopying,
recording, or by any information storage and retrieval system, without permission
in writing from the publisher.

Library of Congress Cataloging-in-Publication Data

Names: Beery, Itzhak, 1950- author.
Title: Shamanic healing : traditional medicine for the modern world /
  Itzhak Beery ; foreword by Alberto Villoldo.
Description: Rochester, Vermont : Destiny Books, [2017] | Includes index.
Identifiers: LCCN 2016048384 (print) | LCCN 2016049832 (e-book) |
  ISBN 9781620553763 (paperback) | ISBN 9781620553770 (e-book)
Subjects: LCSH: Mental healing. | Shamanism. | Mind and body. | BISAC:
  BODY, MIND & SPIRIT / Spirituality / Shamanism. | HEALTH &
  FITNESS / Alternative Therapies.
Classification: LCC RZ999 .B44 2017 (print) | LCC RZ999 (e-book) |
  DDC 615.8/528—dc23
LC record available at https://lccn.loc.gov/2016048384

Printed and bound in the United States by Versa Press, Inc.

10 9 8 7 6 5 4 3 2 1

Text design and layout by Virginia Scott Bowman
This book was typeset in Garamond Premier Pro with Goudy Sans and Hypatia
Sans used as display typefaces

To send correspondence to the author of this book, mail a first-class letter to the
author c/o Inner Traditions • Bear & Company, One Park Street, Rochester, VT
05767, and we will forward the communication, or contact the author directly at
itzhakbeery.com.

To Margalit for the lifelong adventurous journey we embarked on and for Ariel, Tal, and Shira, who make it worthwhile. To Don José Joaquin Piñeda and Bernardo Peixoto, Ph.D., (Ipupiara Makunaiman) for their generous treasured teachings and open hearts.

Contents

Foreword

Alberto Villoldo, Ph.D.

How do you make sense of a magical world infused with energy, spirits, divine beings, restless ancestors, angelic guides, and maleficent forces that can destroy your health?

You can't.

The Western mind is not trained to comprehend the invisible world, the realm that shamans enter in the dreamtime and during waking ceremony in order to heal their clients. And when we can't make sense of something, when it does not fit within our ordinary worldview, we simply determine that it doesn't exist, it cannot exist, because it would shatter our notion of reality.

But our notion of reality is already falling apart all by itself. The reality is that the third leading cause of death in America is hospitals and that if you live to be eighty-five years old you will have a 50 percent chance of having diagnosable Alzheimer's. The reality is that one in forty children is diagnosed with autism today, whereas twenty years ago it was only one in ten thousand. Our mind is making us sick. Chronic stress is wreaking havoc on our immune systems, two of three Americans are overweight or obese, and one of three American children will be diabetic.

Who would have thought . . .

In my early twenties I was a medical anthropologist working in the Amazon basin. At that time the rain forest in central Peru, where the Ucayali River flows into the Amazon, was rife with terrorists and coca plantations. Few foreigners ventured into the area, which was ripe for exploration.

One of my sponsors was a Swiss pharmaceutical giant hoping to find the next big cure for cancer or dementia. After all, the rain forest is nature's pharmacy, replete with herbs, barks, and roots with still-to-be-discovered healing properties.

After months of canoeing to villages that had seldom seen a light-skinned person, I returned to my sponsors empty-handed. In none of the villages that I visited was there any incidence of cancer, heart disease, or dementia. As it turns out, these are the illnesses of civilization, caused by our Western diet, our lifestyle, and our disconnection from nature.

Can the traditional healers from the Amazon and Andes help us repair our bodies and mend our fragmented psyches? You will learn in this book that the answer is yes: that the shamans have a health care system, in sharp contrast to our disease-care system, that they don't treat symptoms only, that they use their tracking skills to find the origin of disease and treat it at its source.

Western medicine practices heal by organ (cardiologists, ophthalmologists, neurologists, etc.) or by disease (oncologists, rheumatologists, etc.). Rarely do the specialists speak with each other. Even though we know that many psychiatric conditions are caused by imbalances in our gut flora, where overpopulation by "bad" microbes releases toxins that cause mood disorders, rarely do GI docs speak with psychiatrists, and the latter seldom if ever recommend probiotics to their patients suffering from anxiety, depression, or mood swings.

Shamans, on the other hand, look on the person as a system, an organism. We are beings of flesh and blood and spirit. We are intrinsically connected to our ancestors, who continue to haunt us or protect us, and to our yet unborn grandchildren. We are part of nature, connected to the forest, the rivers, and the mountains where we live and to the spirits that inhabit these wild places.

The shaman must engage all of these invisible forces and beings when he or she works with a client. And when all of these spiritual forces are brought into balance, then there is a possibility for the client to recover his or her health.

This requires a skilled practitioner who knows the ways of the visible and the invisible world. The shaman must have allies in all three worlds (upper, lower, and middle) and have the strength and courage to occasionally go to battle to rescue or ransom his or her client's soul.

Shamanic training involves many years of studying with skilled teachers and in nature, where the shaman is taught directly by spirit. It is a rigorous training where the shaman learns the art and practice of shamanic healing by embarking on his or her own healing journey—facing demons and befriending them and understanding his or her hidden, shadow side so that the shaman does not project it onto clients or students.

Then there are the lessons of power. Shamans clearly postulate that there is a difference between information and wisdom. Information is understanding that water is H_2O, while wisdom is being able to make it rain. Information is knowing a diagnosis, while wisdom is being able to heal.

Today we are inundated with information: we can find out facts in an instant through our digital devices. Yet we cannot find wisdom in the virtual space more and more of us are inhabiting.

One of the shamans portrayed is a *yachak*. The word comes from the Quechua word *yachay,* meaning "knowledge" or "wisdom" He is a wisdomkeeper. This book is infused with such wisdom.

Itzhak Beery has traveled, studied, and lived with the shamans he writes about. He has gone through a true apprenticeship in the jungles and mountains and has become a shaman in his own right. He has worked with clients who had no hope or prospect for healing.

This book is a guide that can serve many of us who are looking for new ways to live, to grow, and to heal in ways that are sustainable and in right relationship with nature and with spirit. I trust that it will serve as a compass in your own quest for meaning and health in your life.

Alberto Villoldo, Ph.D., is a medical anthropologist who has studied the healing practices of Amazonian and Andean shamans. Villoldo directs the Four Winds

Society, where he trains individuals in the United States and Europe in the practice of shamanic energy medicine. He is the founder of the Light Body School, which has campuses in New York, California, and Germany, where he trains practitioners in energy medicine. He is the author of several books, including *Shaman, Healer, Sage; The Four Insights; Courageous Dreaming;* and *Power Up Your Brain.*

Acknowledgments

To all the medicine men and women by many names throughout the world who have kept this age-old wisdom alive despite the obstacles modern life presented them, there are not enough words to thank you. Thank you for showing us the way to the future.

Deep gratitude to Leah De Santo and especially Glori Anne Di Toro and Meghan MacLean for their hard work in making sense of my manuscript and their honest feedback, which contributed greatly to the final book. To my dear friend Ariel Orr Jordan for continually finding the right words to instigate, inspire, and sharpen this book's vision.

To Ehud Sperling and all the Inner Tradition team for making this book happen. Credit goes to Joe Kulin, my agent, whose guiding hands and friendship I value a great deal.

Thanks to the core members of the New York Shamanic Circle, which I cofounded and whose backing gave me wings to fly on for the last twenty years. A special thank you to all my clients throughout the world: your trust in me taught me more than I could ever imagine possible and mostly about myself and the great mystery.

Finally, I owe deep gratitude to my big-hearted teachers who I was so fortunate to encounter and work with on this long path of healing. Thank you for your faith in me, especially the *yachak* Don José Joaquin Piñeda of Ecuador and the *pajé* Ipupiara Makunaiman of the Brazilian Amazon. Thanks also to Don Alberto Taxo; Don Esteban Tamayo and his two sons, Jorge and Jose; Don Jacho Castilo; Donna Maria Juana and her husband, Don Antonio Yamberla; Don Oscar Santillan; Don Shairy-José Quimbo Pechimba; and Susana Tapia Leon—who all come from the high-energy volcanic-charged Ring of Fire of the Andes of Ecuador. Many thanks also to the Amazonian Shuar's Uwishin Daniel Guachapa, the Inuit uncle Agaangaq Angakkorsuaq, and Native Americans Lewis Mehl-Madrona and Nelson Turtle, along with John Perkins, Hank Wesselman, Michael Harner, Lynn V. Andrews, Nan Moss, David Corbin, and Tom Cowan, who enriched my world beyond words as well. I thank you all.

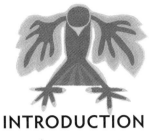

INTRODUCTION
Uniting Shamanic Healing and Western Medicine

Allopathic medicine is a sick-based medicine model. It fails to address the root cause or functional basis of disease. It is treating the smoke, and not the fire.

FRED GROVER JR., M.D., F.A.A.F.P.,
A.B.I.H.M., A.B.A.A.R.M.

To help you navigate and get the most of this book the content was divided into five major chapters.

In this introductory chapter, I argue the inevitable return of the ancient shamanic healing wisdom and the urgent need for shamanic healing and Western medicine to be offered in tandem as a wholesome, healing, and curing solution for our time.

Chapter 1 invites you to meet my teachers and learn about my personal journey. While chapter 2 attempts to explain what shamanic healing is, who can become a shaman, and other information associated with this.

Chapter 3 provides step-by-step instructions on many healing teachings, ceremonies, and techniques, such as La Limpia, diagnostic and divination reading, protection techniques, and additional healing tips for you to use.

And the best, I kept for the last chapter: thirty true and inspiring healing stories, in which the power of miracles, mystery, and ancient know-how changed and healed people's lives.

Read on and enjoy.

◇ ◇ ◇

"I have consulted internists, dermatologists, urologists, psychiatrists, and a neurologist regarding the unexplained sensations and associated pains, but no specialist in any of these fields has found any pathology. I believe that I require soul retrieval and an entity extraction."

So read the e-mail I received, one of many sent by people from all walks of life and professions who have tried conventional medicine without success. Why is it that Western medicine doesn't have the answers and proper treatments for these people? How is it happening that they are "miraculously" healed by practitioners who are trained to use ancient shamanic healing tools? Something must be fatally wrong in the approach we take to health care in our society. The man who wrote me that e-mail received his answers and was healed in a session. How?

Another client wrote, "I don't know why I came to see you in the first place. Maybe I was desperate. I tried lawyers, counselors, and the 'normal' ways. But nothing happened. After each of our sessions something strange happened. After the first one I found pennies everywhere even in places I could not imagine. After the second session I found dimes everywhere, and after the third I found feathers everywhere. Isn't it strange? I think there is magic in what you do. Or maybe my awareness became wider and larger? Yes, I feel so different."

Yes, you could say there is "magic" in traditional shamanic healing. But it only seems like magic in Western society, with its emphasis on rational thinking, scientific proofs, and materialistic consumerism, as we learn to dismiss the metaphysical energy world.

HIT-AND-RUN MEDICINE

I coined this phrase to describe allopathic medicine because of its sick-based model, profit-minded assembly line, speed-dating-like, impersonal human interactions, and the use of medicine by trial-and-error methods.

I sincerely do not fault the individual doctors and their staffs as they are under so much pressure from the corporations and their shareholders. Today, those pressures are rapidly growing with the new capability of digital diagnostic methods and robotic surgery, which may make the work that many of these doctors do obsolete.

Fifty-nine percent of all Americans (188 million people) are taking prescription drugs daily, as recently reported in the *Journal of the American Medical Association,* while 15 percent of all Americans take five drugs or more each day. That is astonishing. Isn't it? Costs and premiums are rising, quality of services are declining. The Anxiety and Depression Association of America notes that 10 percent of Americans are depressed and 18 percent suffer from anxiety. We must and can do better.

The following and surprising story illustrates this point perfectly. One afternoon as I walked into my optometrist's office, a man I did not recognize came out to greet me. I was confused. When I finally recognized his sparkling blue eyes under his fashionable glasses, he had to help close my gaping jaws. "What happened to you? You lost half your weight?" I finally asked him as I caught my breath. He laughed out loud.

"My health was so bad that my doctor wanted to send me for an emergency kidney transplant. I called my brother, who is an alternative doctor. He persuaded me to try a pricy health clinic program in Arizona. I had nothing to lose so I went. On my first day there my assigned doctor asked me to bring all of my medications. I handed him a bag full of thirty-six different prescription medications that I was taking every day. He smiled and threw the bag into the garbage. 'You will not need them anymore,' he said. I was shocked and frightened. 'I'm going to die here,' I thought to myself. 'You see that pole in the middle of this yard? Circle it seven times,' he said. 'Are you out of your mind?' I protested. 'I am 350 pounds. I can hardly walk. I can't breathe,' I begged him. 'Try it,' he said. So I did.

"In just a few weeks my high blood pressure became normal. My diabetes was under control and my kidneys were functioning again; I am pain free and walking three to four miles a day. All without even one pill." He smiled broadly.

Did your doctor ask you how you are feeling? Where you are from, your emotional state, your lifestyle, your social and cultural beliefs, or what you eat? It's not his fault. He did not have the time. He was not trained in medical school to show interest in you. You are just a piece of meat with no soul or spirit attached. There are others to attend to, others to bill. Sound familiar?

Scientific? Not really. Allopathic medicine is based on trial-and-error research. Mostly we know how the body works but not really why. Like my brain scientist friend who asked, "Can you repeat your shamanic journeys three times with the same accurate results?" "No," I replied, "because each person is different." Allopathic medicine may cure or merely mask the symptoms in the afflicted organ while creating unwanted toxic side effects in other organs, which often means that still more medications are needed to treat the side effects, as was so nicely demonstrated by my optometrist's story.

My friend Ariel told me of an unexpected conversation he had with a high-ranking official in the Ecuadorian government, who is an indigenous Quechua. He told me about his elderly mother who constantly complained about having pains throughout her body. Her shoulders hurt. Her back and legs hurt. She was tired and couldn't walk well, eat, or sleep. He pulled some strings and arranged for her to visit a well-known doctor in a prestigious hospital. The doctor spent five minutes with her, gave her a prescription, and sent her away. He did not take any interest in her. He did not care who she was. He didn't ask where she was from or how many children she has.

Disappointed, she went back to her local shaman in her little town. The shaman greeted her warmly and showed her into his healing room, which was decorated with pictures of saints and candles. Familiar smells of oils and *palo santo* filled the air. He called her by her name. He hugged her. He asked her about all the aches and pain and emotional troubles she was having. He asked her about her husband, her children, and grandchildren and asked their names. He listened deeply about her life. She felt loved. She felt she could put her trust in him. The shaman massaged her and performed a healing cleansing ceremony. When she left after two hours, she felt well, hopeful, and pain free. Her heart was happy."

Is allopathic medicine safer than shamanic healing? Let's check the statistics. A 2010 Office of Inspector General for Health and Human Services study concluded that mistakes and infections in hospital care contributed to the deaths of 180,000 patients in Medicare alone in a given year. A recent study of hospital patients in general in the *Journal of Patient Safety* put the numbers much higher: between 210,000 and 440,000 patients each year. Medical errors are the third-leading cause of death in America, behind heart disease and cancer.

Curious to know why some doctors decided to start practicing shamanic healing, I asked Lewis Mehl-Madrona, M.D., Ph.D., from the Eastern Maine Medical Center and Acadia Hospital in Bangor and associate professor, family medicine, University of New England College of Osteopathic Medicine. Here is what he said:

> Having been a practicing physician in the conventional medical system for forty years now, I can celebrate the successes of conventional medicine, which are largely in the area of trauma. However, our obsession with pharmaceuticals is not as successful as I was led to believe in medical school pharmacology class, especially I have also observed that much that we do, does not work, especially for the common miseries of life.
>
> Of course, benzodiazepines reduce anxiety, but then the person becomes addicted and tolerant, and the drugs increase their risk for dementia, which is also problematic. The other medications are only a bit better than placebo in most randomized, controlled trials. In my conventional work, I see a succession of people requesting "the right" medicine for their anxiety. Most of them have good reason to worry. They are disadvantaged economically, out of work, in and out of relationship crises, and generally existentially insecure. In their shoes, I would worry, too.
>
> A traditional, indigenous healer would probably be much more

effective for most of these people. Prayer and ceremony would probably help their anxiety more than fluoxetine and all the other drugs we give them.

This is what today's world needs as an antidote to the greed of *Homo economicus:* the wisdom of the indigenous world for collaboration, cooperation, mutual support, and respect for all of life. This is what the world's traditional, indigenous healers are providing people that conventional medicine is not.

In a personal correspondence, Fred Grover Jr., M.D., F.A.A.F.P., A.B.I.H.M., A.B.A.A.R.M., assistant clinical professor, family medicine, University of Colorado Denver, had even harsher things to say:

I turned to shamanic healing because my traditional allopathic medicine training in family medicine seemed insufficient in treating the deeper causes of disease and mental illness. Allopathic medicine is a sick-based medicine model. It fails to address the root cause or functional basis of disease. It is treating the smoke, and not the fire.

The insurers are interested in providing the least amount of care for their patients to optimize profits back to the CEO and shareholders. Health savings accounts (HSA) offer some hope to cover shamanic healing, but the insurance groups are lobbying to cut HSAs down so that we are forced into the more traditional plans that make them money.

My passion is prevention and wellness, and I couldn't do it with Prozac and Lipitor. I have been blessed with being able to travel the world and explore ancient cultures, see shamans at work, and work with energy medicine healers from many disciplines. This has shifted me energetically and spiritually, which has opened the door to treatment beyond the realms of modern medicine. Being willing to boldly explore shamanistic therapies and trusting in the universe has given me insights that may never be revealed to other physicians. Of course I use a comprehensive history and exam, but adding in intuition has given me a higher degree of accuracy in diagnosis and treatment.

I do hope many will hear their words, and we can move to a more holistic health system.

THE FIRST AND LAST BREATH

There is nothing more telling about the gap between allopathic medicine and shamanic healing than the way they approach the beginning and ending of life. In our intimidating and impersonal hospitals, the pregnant woman is considered sick. She lies in a sterile room and is provided with painkillers to avoid experiencing the pain of birth. According to the U.S. National Center for Health Statistics, 32.2 percent of all women choose to do a costly cesarean section under anesthesia. Rarely are family members allowed to be present to support her. Once the baby is out, he is taken away, separated from his mother, and fed with sugar water.

Indigenous societies celebrate the newborn's arrival with welcoming ceremonies. On one of my trips to Brazil's Rio Negro, I learned about one of those welcoming ceremonies. As our riverboat landed in the small port of a tiny town on the river, I spotted a small store selling the native arts and craft of the Waimiri-Atroari. One of the items that caught my eyes was a beautiful brown and white woven hammock made of *swita,* a special strong river grass. I opened it up, and to my surprise there was a big hole in the middle of it. I asked the young, native attendant why the hammock was made this way.

"Oh, this is a birthing hammock," she giggled as she saw my confused face. "When the woman is ready to give birth, her family hangs this hammock between two trees and digs a deep hole in the earth below. The woman sits in the hammock, positioning her vulva over the hammock opening. When the baby comes out, before they clean him up, he is lowered into the hole to be greeted by Mother Earth first. He is then given to his human mother to be breastfed. Then her nutrient-rich placenta is buried in the pit, connecting the two mothers and enriching the earth." During all of this, a group of women celebrate the arrival of the new member of the community. What a remarkable difference.

There is also a big difference in how indigenous people deal with death versus modern Western society. In the Uru-e-wau-wau Amazonian tribe tradition according to Ipupiara, my mentor, after a person has passed on, the body is burned on an open fire pit as the family and community watch and pray for a smooth transition into the spirit world. After the body is reduced to ashes, the bones are crushed into a fine powder and put in a big bowl. They mix it with water until it becomes like a soup, and in a ceremonial manner each of the family members in turn ingests a small amount of it. In this way the ancestor becomes an integral part of each of them and continues to live in and through them forever. Imagine, every one of them carries all their ancestors memories for eternity in an unbroken chain. Once the ceremony is complete, it is forbidden to grieve and mention the deceased's name. Of course Western ways are very different.

WESTERN MEDICINE
VERSUS SHAMANIC HEALING

Should we use the gifts of the relatively new technologies of Western medicine? The answer is a resounding yes. There could be great benefits by integrating both technologies and using them in tandem. According to the National Institutes of Health research, almost 40 percent of adult Americans (about 120 million) are regularly using complementary alternative medicine today. They are looking for other options. Searching for healing methods that better support their lifestyles and belief systems to heal not just the body but the mind and the spirit as well.

A few years ago, by complete chance, I discovered, by standing in front of an ionizing machine (an alternative healing method) that I had three large cancerous tumors sitting on top of my thyroid. This explained why my voice had become hoarse and why I had two Adam's apples in my neck. I was shocked and desperate. Why me? Why now? What had I done to deserve this? I battled with myself perpetually: Should I resort to shamanic methods and ask my teachers to heal me, or should I go the allopathic route? I strongly believed that I had to walk the walk and be an example to my clients. But my shamanic teachers unequivocally recommended that I immediately undergo surgery and have the tumors removed. And so I did, and I am grateful for my competent surgeon and his latest technology. But it was the shamanic healing ceremony I received prior to the surgery that gave me the emotional peace of mind to go through the procedure and helped me recover faster. Ironically, the cancer I had was caused by external radiation treatment I went through many years ago to cure small acne on my nose.

If a doctor or healer takes into consideration a patient's emotional state and cultural and spiritual beliefs, the patient will most likely experience less stress and resistance and will be more ready to accept treatment, thus increasing the chances for a more complete recovery. I have shared this belief with many medical doctors and psychologists who themselves have come to me for treatments and have recommended shamanic healing to their clients.

Today, with new awareness, many doctors and medical facilities are offering what we call alternative modalities on their premises, such as reiki, reflexology, acupuncture, and more, or recommend it to their clients. Thus the new term *integrative medicine* has emerged, which takes into account the whole client, his or her lifestyle, belief system, mind, body, and spirit.

I know of other shamans who will recommend their clients to see a doctor or have a surgery done. I do hope that soon shamanic healing will be offered in the hospitals as one of their treatment options and will someday be covered by health insurance.

For instance, Ipupiara, a Brazilian shaman, was asked to perform his tradition of shamanic healing ceremonies in a Washington, D.C., cancer hospital. He reported enthusiastically that the bodies of the people he worked on responded better to chemotherapy and recovered faster than those who did not receive his treatment. "Calming and balancing the physical and emotional bodies creates less opposition for the medicine, which allows it to work better," he told me.

I myself have had the privilege of holding healing ceremonies for my clients in hospitals where they were receiving treatment or even in hospice care, always in agreement with the care staff. Sometimes the family was present to witness the ceremony. I could see the positive results immediately.

When I performed a cleansing ceremony for my dying friend Joyce while she lay in her hospital bed, she later felt so relaxed that she did not need the morphine she was using until the next morning. Her mood changed, and the anger and fear she was consumed by were replaced by genuine acceptance of her final journey. It was a gift for her and her anxious family.

Just a few hours before another client's major liver transplant surgery in a prestigious hospital in Manhattan, as the head of the ICU department watched the door, I performed a cleansing ceremony for her. This young woman was obviously anxious and in deep panic, as there was a good chance her body would reject the new organ and the surgery would fail. I needed her help, so I suggested we simultaneously connect to our spirit guides during the ceremony. I asked her to connect to her power animal and ask it to bring her to meet the power of Imbabura Mountain, a volcanic mountain in Ecuador, and embody his strength and grounding into her weakening body. At the same time, in the spirit world, I quickly connected to an indigenous island woman whom I had discovered a few days earlier in a separate vision requested by my client's mother, and the details of which were confirmed by my client. Standing at the entrance of a small house by a small hotel, protected by the early evening darkness and the surrounding trees, this indigenous woman had cursed my client, who had just arrived in Bali with a friend. That curse, spirit said, had brought this horrible liver failure on her quite immediately.

I pleaded with the long-dark-haired, angry, short woman to release this young girl who laid here in the hospital bed from her horrible curse. She did not relent easily, but I begged her, telling her that my client was the only child of loving parents—just like her own daughter—and that she meant the whole world to them.

The girl could not be blamed for the woman's marital and economic troubles, caused, as she believed, by Western visitors to the island. After a while, I could see her anger cracking and transforming into compassion. She apologized for her misdirected anger. I commended her on her great magical power and asked her to use it for my client's benefit by sending good healing energy to her before the upcoming operation. I watched that woman making her prayers, moving her hands up and down and forward, far away in Bali, and then she disappeared. At the end of the ceremony I blew my ocarina close to my client's resting head and she opened her eyes and smiled. "I feel calm and ready for the operation. I'm going to take the mountain with me," she said. I shared with her my exchange vision with that native woman she knew. "Thank you. I needed that," she smiled. The operation was a success.

Contrary to some people's beliefs, shamanic healing or shamanism is not a spiritual practice in itself. It is a very result-oriented system that uses many tools to induce positive changes in a person's life. One of the tools used is working directly with spirits. And believe me, if a shaman sees that one tool he uses won't do the job, he will exchange it in favor of one that does. A shaman's reputation solely depends on the actual results of his healing work.

Maybe the difference between these two systems can be described in this way: like a gardener, Western medicine attempts to clear the weeds from the garden by spraying chemicals or nipping the leaves and stems above the surface. The shamanic healer, by contrast, searches for the emotional and spiritual roots of the illness and pulls them out from the ground.

Poor health, disease, dysfunction, and depression are signs that the client is out of alignment. That explains the experience of many clients of mine who report, after shamanic ceremonial healing sessions, unexpected positive results, such as better, more restful sleep, clearer thinking, feeling more grounded, and improved digestion. They also report being able to stop smoking, find they no longer get migraine headaches, and so much more.

IS IT ONLY A PLACEBO EFFECT OR THEATER?

"Oh, it's just hocus-pocus or theater—the placebo effect. I'd rather just take a pill and that's that." I've been told this many times by skeptical people from all walks of life, implying that shamanic healing has no real healing value.

"What's wrong with that?" I always reply. A number of double-blind scientific studies have proved again and again that a test group given sugar pills will experience as much pain relief as the group given a pain reliever. So why take a chemical if your own mind can heal your body and emotions? Both the shaman and the Western doctor use a certain amount of theater to gain their clients' trust and confidence. Think of it: both practitioners wear special attire, set up a special environment that has special ambience, and perform rituals with special tools.

I believe that the rituals, ceremonies, and storytelling of indigenous shamanic traditions are the foundation and inspiration for what we call theater and are used essentially as a tool for personal and large-scale community healing. I witnessed this firsthand in the Guatemala highlands during the December 21, 2012, completion celebration of the thirteenth *baktun*—a four-hundred-year period of the Mayan calendar and the beginning of the new calendar's cycle.

Don Tómas Calvo, the esteemed K'iche's spiritual leader—whom I had met a few months earlier in New York City—wished to document these rare ceremonies, which happen every 63,080,082 years. I was asked to be the shamanic consultant for the film crew by my friend Tucker Robbins.

The elaborate ceremonies were beautifully set in the middle of Chichicastenango's large town square. It was bracketed on two sides by two old churches—built over an ancient Mayan sun temple in the east and moon temple in the west (as was customary by the Spanish conquerors)—and by many small bodegas selling arts and crafts and local foods. For twenty-four hours, groups of K'iches shamans, children, men, and women who came from throughout the land, dressed in their best traditional colorful ceremonial outfits, shape-shifted and brought to life their twenty *naguals* (the sacred guardian spirits in animal form such as jaguars, pumas, serpents, dogs, birds, bats, coyotes, etc., who it is believed accompany and guide humans). They shared the universe creation stories and other tribal wisdom. It was one of the most moving events I have ever experienced. I entered a pure, infinite, dreamlike world that transcended the limitations of time and space.

Quietly and in awe, I stood in the midst of the large multilayered circles of hundreds of locals, along with some tourists. At two in the morning, at the last ceremony before the new baktun began at sunrise, the strong voice of the master of ceremonies came through the loudspeakers as he engaged the audience by narrating their creation story. All the while repetitive hypnotic marimba and xylophone rhythms helped us all enter into a deep trance. Clouds of thick dark smoke covered the entire square, rising to the stars from many multicolored candles and from big copal balls that were put into the five large bonfires, one for each of the four directions and one for the center, which represents our heart. The strong distinctive scent of the copal resin filled the chilly night air and our nostrils. Moving rhythmically in circles, some of the participants offered the bonfires devotional prayers and asked personal questions and for guidance. They stopped, stared into the flames, observing the patterns and colors—flickers of light snaking up to the dark skies—and waited for answers. Others moved from one bonfire to the next to stoke them, breathing life into them. Dancers dressed as the twenty naguals with colorful and imaginative masks brought those entities into life, moving with surprising agility and natural grace from one side of the square to the other as the marimba continued its endless loop. And then it happened. For a few moments time stopped. I found myself losing my grip on the square's cobblestones and I was ascending, transported into an infinite mystical reality that had no beginning and no end, floating in eternity, connecting to the mystery and matrix of life itself. Somehow I snapped out of it and noticed the silent audience, both young and old, seemed wholly transfixed and immersed in the unfolding saga as they followed the teachings of their calendar, deities, and heritage. Looking at their intense glowing faces, I also sensed that they gained affirmation and pride in their indigenous culture and self-identity. They were recovering and healing from thirty-six years (1960–1996) of brutal civil war, which was supported by the United States, and which was started to protect United Fruit Company lands from being nationalized. Two hundred thousand native peoples were killed as terrorists or guerillas.

As the sun slowly rose in the east above the town's cemetery and painted the early morning sky with passionate shades of reds, oranges, and yellows, the ceremony ended. It was time for welcoming the new baktun in a newly built plaza behind the cemetery. I quickly found myself marching with the big crowd, as if someone ordered us down the steep hill. A small group of drummers and musicians were playing their musical instruments loudly in the front, leading the way. Loud "boombas" exploded now and again to let the community know to join the parade. When we reached the bottom of the steep hill we started climbing up again into the cemetery full of multicolored painted tombs. As we passed among the long rows of graves the locals stopped to pay respect to their ancestors. Truly, a mesmerizing collective healing materialized.

There is plenty of scientific research today that proves without any doubt that the mind, body, and spirit connection is responsible for creating demonstrable physical changes in our physical and emotional bodies on a cellular, DNA, and hormonal level for humans and perhaps for other animals and plants too.

Both shamanic and theater practices aspire to circumvent our skeptical, cynical, and critical logical mind—our gatekeeper—by creating a sacred nonordinary space and reality in which our physical reality and our belief systems can be challenged and transcended. This is achieved through the creative use of emotional, nonverbal symbols and sensual, engaging narrative. Storytelling can be amplified by special effects, lighting, and enticing decorations and through the voices, songs, and instrumental sounds. In both the main characters are hiding themselves behind animal or human masks or painted faces while wearing special costumes. Doing this enables us to challenge and transcend our limiting physical world and belief systems and enter a time and space where everything is possible. A magical transformation happens and all our senses are enlivened, including that mysterious "sixth sense" of vision and knowing.

WHY SHAMANIC HEALING IS RELEVANT TODAY

I hope when you finish reading this book you will fully understand and even demand that these ancient healing methods should be fully embraced by our Western society and be covered by health providers and insurance companies. You will read more stories like that in the following pages. But first, what is shamanic healing, and how does it work?

Indigenous people the world over have kept shamanic healing methods and perspectives alive for many thousands of years. Frequently, the carriers of these precious practices struggled to keep them alive, as their cultures and people were being conquered, outlawed, burned, and persecuted by more "technologically advanced" civilizations, which destroyed their temples, sacred places, and heritage. In an effort to preserve that heritage, practices, rituals, and customs were hidden in faraway hard-to-reach corners of Earth and practiced in the thick of night, in the depths of caves, or hidden at the top of remote mountains. These secrets were passed verbally from mother to daughter and from grandfather to grandchild for generations. Within our own Western cultures this wisdom was often hidden and buried in the texts of fairytales and lullabies as well as in religious symbols and rituals. They were also kept as countless superstitious beliefs and grandmother's tales. In the past few thousand years, the three major monotheistic religions—Judaism, Christianity, and Islam—forbade them and punished women who practiced them, sometimes by even burning them alive. We owe a debt of tremendous gratitude to all our ancestors who so dutifully carried this wisdom to our modern-day digital generation.

Shamanic healing returns us to the core principles of healthiness and a balanced life by using the gifts of Earth and those of the spirit world. It brings us in contact with all our senses and develops them, especially the sixth sense, which lets us connect to the unseen world and our intuition. With the proliferation of smart phones and other electronic gadgets, our brain more and more relies on them, making us more dependent and, yes, lazy. I call it "the Big Shutdown of the Senses," as all the answers and information we are looking for are now easily available through gadgets. We have become less and less observant of and engaged in the world around us. For example, these gadgets "free" us from having to orient ourselves on Earth by the four directions in order to reach our destination: we just follow Waze, Google Maps, or what Siri tells us. We can learn time of the day and the weather by consulting the Internet or an app instead of observing the sky and wind. We don't have to remember phone numbers, know much math, or memorize history or geography facts. We don't even have to know how we feel or listen to our bodies; there are apps that do that too. Smart devices create a virtual reality and virtual communities on one small flat screen.

Shamanic healing returns us to personally experiencing our all-encompassing relationship with the universe and the true reason why we are here. Above all, it makes possible the survival of the human race on this miraculous planet we all share.

But before we start, here is a courtesy warning: what you are about to read is written from my collected and scattered personal notebooks, from my subjective memory, and from my accumulated and personal work experiences. As I am sure you well know, memories can be very fluid. Two people who take part in the same event describe it in two different ways and from two different points of views. For this reason, I have not included a bibliography, notes, or resources at the end of this book.

I hope that you will allow yourself to experience my stories with all of your senses. I assume it will require a considerable leap of faith. It is my modest personal journey and life experience, and by all means, I invite you to disagree or even prove me wrong. I am sure some of my teachers would say that they never meant or said this or that, or that I misunderstood what they said. It is possible; it is the nature of shamanism. It is an ever-changing personal journey of each individual shaman, sometimes contradictory, as is the nature of the world itself. Time and time again, my teachers would change the strict explicit instructions they gave me and would instead "improvise," as the spirit instructed them at a particular moment and under the conditions that were presented to them. One teacher said, "Spirit told me to . . . ," while another told me, "There is no right or wrong; it is in spirit's hands," which sometimes left me, of course, puzzled.

To keep the reading flowing and interesting, I have tried to write the book through adventures and storytelling from which the reader can extract the techniques and teaching. The generous teachings, which I am attempting to share with you, came mainly from my two teachers. Additionally I took some liberty to incorporate my other teachers' teachings into the stories as well.

Shamanism has become a mainstream cultural buzzword in recent years. It's truly everywhere you turn your head to, from hit movies to video and computer games and the music industry. Bookshelves are exploding with new titles for adults and children in the shamanic category. Magazine and newspaper articles abound; even mainstream-media-sensationalizing celebrities seek shamanic healing. Soccer teams and politicians call on shamans to help them win. New forms of shamanism are now popping up everywhere: shamanic yoga, shamanic reiki, shamanic trance dance, shamanic breath work, and shamanic astrology are just a few examples of this trend. Shamanic seminars, teachings, and adventure trips to faraway exotic places are plentiful and growing, and if you search the word *shamanism* on the Internet, you will see millions of entries. You might ask yourself, "What's going on here, and why now?" There are many very good reasons.

The shamanic worldview is an antithesis to our Western industrious, scientific mind culture's teaching, which celebrates and rewards separateness of the human race and the superiority of the individualist—exemplified by Ayn Rand's writings—over the well-being of the whole community, vilifying codependency. Worldview that admires scientific brain power and control over nature and weather and of other people, worldview that sees success in accumulation of personal resources, wealth, and property, that values competition and lives in fear of scarcity, worldview that encourage a person to follow orders of governments, corporations, or dogmatic religious teachings.

Indigenous societies, however, hold the belief that the Great Creator, that great mysterious force that has no form or gender, created all there is for a reason, sometime unbeknown to us. Thus everything in our world is sacred and one and the same. In other words, humans are not superior in nature's pecking order to other animals or the environment and thus should not have dominion over nature. They believe in interdependency; they believe in living in harmony with nature and sharing Earth's abundance of resources without private ownership of the land. They believe people should experience and practice as their own spirits direct them.

My main realization when I first visited the rain forest was that every plant couldn't grow without its supporting neighboring plants. Every animal serves a unique purpose to the whole ecology of the jungle, just as the jungle has a special relationship to Earth. If you remove a single plant or animal, the whole environment around it collapses. We truly are all interdependent.

The scientific and technological innovations of the past decades have brought about globalization, which has brought us closer together. Through satellite connections and the World Wide Web, we can reach almost every corner of the world; city and jungle dwellers can meet and exchange information instantly. People deep in jungles or on the tops of high mountains are exposed to Western ideas, music, fashion, and technological innovations.

We too are now able to comprehend and appreciate indigenous societies' age-old wisdom, simple practicality, and stewardship of Earth. Within the diversity of their traditions we can find an outline for our own well-being and survival. Recognizing that although we have almost everything we need in our materialistic world, we are missing a deeper connection to our primal roots of the natural world and to our own nature. I believe we are all souls who yearn to be one, to reunite with all of nature again. Additionally, I feel, as many in our society do, an uneasy feeling that many questions about our current life complexities are not being answered by technology, mainstream religions, and institutions, which are failing to address and offer real solutions.

Interestingly, two trends are happening simultaneously. In the West, since the 1960s, people like Michael Harner, Hank Wesselman, and John Perkins, who were sent by the Peace Corps or their universities into the jungles of South America, Africa, or Asia, have been attracting people with their stories, books, and teachings, including myself. By studying with them, we discover that we can trust the unknown, our own powerful connection to the natural forces, and our ability to interact with those forces, as well as the importance of supportive communities. At the same time, following their ancient prophecies' teaching of the arrival of new era of collaboration among all people on Earth, many shamans are coming out of hiding. They hear the call to share with us in the Western world their secrets, which have kept those societies alive from beginning of time.

What can be the benefits of shamanism for you? Spiritual, emotional, and physical healing are common benefits in the shamanic practice. It releases anxiety and stress, eases loneliness, and restores faith and the physical body's vigor. Shamans view illness as caused by falling out of balance and being separated and disconnected from nature and one's family and community.

Shamanism offers its practitioners an alternative way of life, personal empowerment, and a kindhearted community. Shamanism's nonverbal communication methods seep deeply into one's soul, activating the primary forces that trigger all of our senses. It helps us get in touch with our own dreams, magic, and mystery. Shamanism is a way to look at what's going on around us and make sense of it without fear, guilt, or shame. As Lynn Andrews said, "Bring chaos into balance." It's a way to live in inner balance and connected to the matrix of life. It's also an opportunity to create personal and community rituals and ceremonies for each stage of our lives.

So how can you bring shamanism into your life? You can read a book or an article on the Internet, take part in a workshop, or experience shamanic healing. But most importantly, start by going to the source. Nature. Observe its life cycle and its flow. Learn to revere and celebrate nature and the environment around you. Go outside of your sheltered life. Worship every blade of grass. Find a tree that is "calling" you and hug it. Close your eyes, listen to the birds calling you, and breathe in deeply. Form a connection with the tree. Feel the interconnectedness that flows between you and the entire universe. Feel your body as the tree trunk. Feel your legs turning into roots, deepening into the earth, pulling in nutrition and energy from Earth's core. Feel your hair becoming the tree leaves and branches fed by the heat of the sun. Feel how you are becoming a bridge between heaven and Earth, between Father Sun and Mother Earth. Feel the connection between you and all other trees. Now, ask the tree a personal question and wait for an answer. I do it often, and I'm always amazed by the wisdom and insights I receive.

I'm sure that you'll feel self-conscious doing that, afraid your friends and family might think you are a bit weird, which reminds me of a story my mentor Ipupiara once told me.

"Every morning my wife and I went to one of Washington, D.C.'s parks to hug a tree, in a simple honoring ceremony. One morning, a young boy of a family that also used to come at the same hour saw us performing our ritual. The boy spontaneously ran toward us and asked me curiously, 'Uncle, what are you doing, why are you hugging these trees?'

"With great patience I explained to the boy, 'You see, trees are living beings too, just like you are. Trees, through their branches and leaves, connect to the sky—the heavens, the sun, the stars—and with Mother Earth. They are holding the world together.' And I showed him with my hands and my feet. 'When we hug them we become connected to the whole world, and we don't feel alone. Each tree has its own personality: some bear fruits; some do not. Some are green all year long, some shed their leaves in the fall, some have deep roots, and some are shallow. Some are tall, some are short, just like people.' And then I asked him, 'Do you know that trees can talk to each other through their leaves and roots?' The boy looked at me with surprise in his big eyes. 'You can speak to them too, and they will understand and send your prayers. Here, touch this tree. Hug it. Can you feel its energy?'

"The boy stretched his small arms around the tree and hugged it strongly, and then with a big smile on his face, he nodded his head up and down for yes! Then without saying good-bye he ran to share his experience with his watching family.

"You wouldn't believe what happened next," Ipupiara said with a smirk in his eyes. "A few days later the whole family came toward us. 'We saw you hugging trees for a few weeks now. Can we participate in your strange ceremony too?' the father asked. I gladly invited them to choose a personal tree for each one of them. In the following days more people joined in until a few months later, we had a regular group of tree huggers. It was so beautiful."

You can agree with me that Ipupiara showed courage and determination. By connecting with nature, following his heart, and feeding his soul through a simple ritual, he created a loving and supportive community of former strangers. That is why ancient shamanism is so relevant today.

WHEN WAS SHAMANISM INVENTED?

No one person can take credit for shamanism; it is the culmination of many traditions and cultures. Shamanic healing has been carried out continuously ever since the beginning of the human race on this planet on every continent. Various people, such as designated healers, men, women, mothers, wives, and even priests, have used it in every community. The proof for its astounding success and resiliency is our own existence today. For all those hundreds of thousands of years of enduring natural disasters and disease, humans did not use aspirin pills, antibiotics, immunization shots, and other modern methods, discoveries that are less then two to three hundred years old. But we still gloriously survived as a species. You can see proof of shamanic healing practices in cave paintings and ancient burial grounds all around the globe.

Near the beginning of the Renaissance in Italy around 1220, the first medical university opened in Siena. I was fortunate to visit that institution a few years ago while teaching a shamanic seminar in Tuscany and saw how they treated their patients. In the United States, the first hospital was Pennsylvania Hospital, which opened in 1751. Prescription drugs were only invented around 1890 with the introduction first of heroin and then aspirin. Only in the nineteenth century did Western medicine, as we know it today, become the norm. From one perspective, Western medicine is actually the new "alternative" medicine compared to age-old shamanic healing.

Every culture around the world developed its own unique healing system in conjunction with its climate, geography, mythology, and stories, using special chants and prayers to go with it. They used their own local natural herbs and minerals and worked with animals and spirits. Sometimes even within a community different family traditions developed. But as a whole the shamanic healing principles are consistent. The belief is that everything in the universe is alive and vibrating with conscious energy and that there is an unseen world and seen world that interact with each other. Shamanic healing is about returning the physical body, spirit, and soul back into balance and harmony.

KEEPER OF THE FIRE

Shaman is a relatively new word. It originates with the Tungus people of Eastern Siberia, a nomadic tribe of hunter-gatherers that spread across the taiga's vast land. In the seventeenth century as the Russian empire reached them, Russians adopted the Tungus word *saman* (the *s* pronounced as *sh*), which described their healers. The word eventually took hold worldwide.

Shaman may mean "one who sees in the dark" or "miracle worker" or "one who knows." Other translations are "one who can fly" or "messenger between the worlds." The definition varies depending on which of the shaman's abilities are being described—for example, the ability to fly or the shaman's role as the go-between of the spirit world and our world. There is no exact translation as there is no exact definition of what a shaman is.

Shaman has become a generic word just as *aspirin,* originally a Bayer trademark name, is now used to describe all medications with acetylsalicylic acid or *google* for all searches on the Internet. It is now a universally recognized term to describe all men or women who are employing traditional folk medicine, natural medicine from Earth, or spirit. There are as many names for this vocation as there are tribes and languages, and some cultures have different names for male and female shamans. Using the word *shaman* for all people who practice this medicine has its benefits, as it has transformed the derogatory connotations many Western cultures and organized religions have stamped on witchcraft and witches, sorcerers, faith healers, and pagans since the Middle Ages in an effort to eradicate ancient spiritual traditions and replace them with the new church doctrines and hegemony. Today, the word *shaman* is used in the furthest places on Earth, in the Amazon and on the high mountains. Even traditional healers have started to call themselves shamans. Maybe it is a sign we are becoming one small village.

Some years ago, I was invited to a special healing ceremony held by an elder Tungus shaman in full attire in a New Jersey private house. It was packed with a diverse group of people, mostly Russian speaking. At the end of this remarkable evening, which truly transported me to the shaman's distant land, I gathered the courage to ask him for the true definition of the word *shaman* in his language. His translator, an elderly Russian anthropology professor, replied briskly, "The keeper of the fire," and turned his back on me. I was surprised; I wasn't expecting to hear that—and also taken aback, wondering if he just wanted to get rid of me. But although this definition was not what I had been told nor had read in many sources, it made a lot of sense and broadened the definition of the shaman—as a person of service, the keeper of the community's soul and well-being.

Although a shaman has many roles in his community—teacher,

healer, and bridge between the seen and unseen worlds—his central role is to be responsible for the physical and spiritual health of his community. He is in charge of keeping the sacred fire, the burning embers, if you wish, of his community's life going. Literally and symbolically, we see fire as a symbol of the source of life. Fire is the principal element that brings warmth, energy, and passion and provides survival or destruction for the community. It is around the sacred fire that, during dark nights, the entire community gathers to hear their ancestors' stories, to hear myths, to sing songs, and to celebrate their togetherness. As keeper of the fire the shaman has a broad and important role as a community sustainer; needless to say, a shaman needs the community as much as the community needs his services. It puts the community at the core of any individual life. Shamanism isn't about individual powers; it's about the strength of the community.

Today we are enjoying a rebirth of shamanic practices exactly because of the destruction of the family unit and the high mobility of people who are yearning to be part of a supportive community.

1

My Journey and Those Who Guided Me

My unexpected journey to becoming a shamanic practitioner started entirely by coincidence, or maybe it was fate, in the summer of 1995. Maybe my great-grandfather had something to do with it, as he was himself a healer and a kabbalistic rabbi in Poland—though I did not learn this until many years later when I taught in Poland myself.

By 1995, I was in my midforties, and as happens to many people, I was in the thick of a midlife crisis. I told myself I should be satisfied with my life, but I wasn't. In my mind, I knew I had achieved quite a bit at this stage of my life, but something huge was missing. There was a big fat void. Many years prior I had left my birthplace, a remote Israeli kibbutz—a collective farming community—and moved to the big city to pursue my visual arts passion and even had an art representative selling my art. I was married to an amazing and talented woman whom I had met in high school and who became the most inspiring dancer. We had migrated to New York City to study and further our art careers. I studied art, exhibited, and at the same time owned a design-advertising agency and worked with both large and small companies. I won many awards for TV and radio commercials, some of which I also directed. I created many cutting-edge and successful print campaigns, which were quite memorable. I helped my wife raise three truly outstanding children. I also believed that I took care of myself. I participated in a self-help group and in a men's support group for almost fifteen years. I took hand-reading and authentic movement workshops. And then I hit a wall: Who am I? Is this all there is for me on this Earth? Why am I here? What will the rest of my life look like? Those were some of the many questions that were constantly tormenting me.

In the summer of 1995, my friend Leighton from my men's support group (the Urban Gorillas) suggested I come with him to a men's retreat in Kalani, on the Big Island of Hawaii. Somehow, by coincidence or fate, the funds appeared from a human angel and I joined him. To pass the time on the long flight from New York City, I needed a book. I rushed to a bookstore minutes before the car took me to the airport, and my eyes caught sight of, by coincidence or fate, a thrilling book—*Spiritwalker* by Hank Wesselman. As I read through it, I started to get some answers to the questions I had been asking myself. I was amazed and thrilled. In the book Wesselman mentioned a workshop he took with an anthropologist, Michael Harner, Ph.D. A few months after returning to New York from my trip to Kalani, Hawaii, I happened to open the New York Open Center's course catalog, and lo and behold, Michael Harner was giving a basic shamanic workshop. Was it a coincidence? I signed up for the workshop. The visionary experiences I had were totally surprising in their material world accuracy and undeniable. I wanted more.

THE TRIP TO ECUADOR THAT CHANGED MY LIFE

Following my experience with Harner, on the spur of the moment and on a suggestion from my friend Ariel, I decided to participate in a workshop given by John Perkins, cofounder of Dream Change Coalition (a nonprofit organization to help raise humanity's consciousness and inspire new ways of living). I did not know who he was, nor had I read his books. I did not know then that my future teacher, Don José, had been one of his teachers, which I would find out years later (Perkins wrote about his apprenticeship in his book *The World Is as You Dream It*). Perkins's incisive environmental message, heartwarming teachings, personal stories, unbounded charisma, and overflowing enthusiasm resonated with me deeply and do even more today.

After the workshop, Perkins, a tall man with a full head of curly hair and winning smile, conducted a fire ceremony. More than twenty men and women in all shapes and ages took their clothes off and walked naked in a circle chanting. John, with a bottle of *trago* (sugarcane rum) in one hand and a lit white candle in the other, blew a cloud of fire (*focay*) over our bare bodies. It was a purifying and exhilarating experience, playful and pleasurable. I did not feel ashamed or self-conscious. Instead, I felt complete freedom, a connection to everything, and unexplained childlike joy.

The next day during the closing ceremony, Perkins told the group that he would be leading a new group to Ecuador soon to meet with the shamans of the Andes and Amazon basin in Orienté. At that moment, I knew I had to go. I did not know why, but it was as if nothing mattered and I had to follow my gut feeling. This decision was against all odds as I did not have the money or the time, and I was burdened by heavy responsibilities to my family and my employees. "Why do you have to go? We can't afford it," my wife rightly said. "I don't know. I only know that I have to," I replied. I felt irresponsible, selfish, guilty, and utterly excited at the same time.

So in March 1997, I joined Perkins with two of my closest friends and a group of curious men and women (mostly healers and psychotherapists) on my first trip to the Ecuadorian Andes and Amazon. During that trip, I met and had my first healing session with the renowned and powerful *yachak* Don José Joaquin Diaz Piñeda. This happened by coincidence, as well, or fate, as Don José was not part of our trip's agenda. Because four of us arrived in Ecuador a few days before the official trip began, we were able to meet Don José, the man who would change my life forever. Don José was one of the shamans on a list that our local tour guide, Juan Gabriel, had given to Juan Carlos, our driver, guide, and interpreter. In another one of many coincidences, I had dreamed about Juan Carlos as our tour guide a few weeks before that trip and we continue to work together till this day, twenty years later.

MEETING DON JOSÉ

Don José Joaquin Diaz Piñeda stood proudly before us, wearing a colorful feather crown, a blue llama wool poncho, and white fabric sandals. He was a short, solid man in his late forties with a high forehead and almond-shaped dark, piercing eyes. His face was smooth and round, darkened by the Andes sun; he had high chiseled cheekbones, and a long braid of jet-black hair hung down his back. He opened the ceremony by blowing trago to the four directions. He closed his eyes and called the power of his mountain's allies with a beautiful ancient chant. He then introduced himself to the participants in Spanish mixed with Quechua:

"I'm José Joaquin Diaz Piñeda. I'm a yachak, which means 'birdman' in my language of Quechua, a wise person who knows how to fly to the other worlds, like a bird. I was born in San Juan de Iluman near Otavalo, the capital of our Imbabura region. I am a member of the Yachak Association of Iluman and have certification from the Ecuadorian government. Yachakuna is an old tradition of our village, and we are very famous all over the world because we use the combined spiritual power of the three powerful volcanic mountains—Imbabura, Cotacachi, and Mojanda—together."

He surveyed us with his sharp eyes, as he waited to be translated.

"I am like a doctor; I heal everyone and everything with plants and ceremonies. I have practiced healing since I was fourteen years old. I come from a long line of yachaks, five generations. I learned it from my grandfather and my father since I was three years old. First they took me to the springs, lakes, and waterfalls to get acquainted with their energies, then to work with fire, air, and earth. Some of my brothers are also yachaks. My work is very well known; I have healed many people, even government officials, judges, generals, and politicians. People come to me from Colombia and other countries, from America, Europe, and South America. Even other shamans from different communities come to see me when they need removal of evil spirits sent to them by other shamans.

"I walk only *el camino illuminoso,* the path of light, which is the yachak path. It is very important to follow the light of your heart, not the temptation of the dark side, because that energy will come back to hurt you."

He looked around the room to see if we understood as he was being translated into English.

THE HEALING CEREMONY

What's going on with me? What is he doing to me? I wondered. A blur of frantic thoughts flooded my mind as a heavy pressure mounted at the center of my forehead. I was one of the first to step forward to undergo the healing ceremony with Don José. He started by having me rub a white candle over my body, which he then lit and examined, and then he blew trago on me from all directions, brushed me with bunch of aromatic green leaves, and began brushing eggs over me while chanting his mesmerizing *icaro*.

I took a big breath and released my fear. In my mind's eye a vision appeared as if a window in space and time had just opened. Through this opening, glowing rays of bright white sunlight poured out to lead me on to perceive a stunning fertile valley dotted with different shades of green. Tall and impressive mountains bounded the valley, as three waterfalls flowed down magically into the valley below. A dazzling large rainbow rose over those lush mountains.

Where am I? What's going on? Is it real? These thoughts rushed through my mind as I felt Don José brushing the eggs over me. A sense of true connection and genuine inner peace with all that surrounded me overcame me. I was surprised. Tears were flowing down my face. Engrossed with the unexpected vision, I did not hear Don José's chants nor did I care. A sharp birdlike whistling behind my neck shook me to alertness, and I slowly opened my eyes. I gasped for air.

What just happened? I felt that something big and important had just ensued, and I did not have the right words to explain it to myself.

The only thing I did know was that I was not the same person who had walked into the room twenty minutes earlier. I felt lighter, as if a ton of weight had lifted off me and a primal secret was revealed to me. I was truly confused.

"Can I hug you now?" Don José asked with a slight smile. We hugged.

"Gracias," I thanked him. He looked at me sternly with his piercing eyes under his colorful feather crown and said, "You need to take a few baths when you go home. Start on Monday, and then Tuesday and Wednesday, and then do the same for the next two weeks." He dictated a list of plants and flowers that I would need to use with full instructions. Juan Carlos scribbled them down on a piece of paper. I put my clothes on and tucked the paper in my pocket. (To my dismay I lost it on our trip to the Shuar tribe in the Amazon.) I slowly sat down on the old wooden bench along the wall of the simple room that was still under construction.

In a daze, I watched my friend undress, preparing to take my place in the center of the room for his healing ceremony. I watched Don José clear the healing plants off the floor and throw them to the left corner, purify his hands with Agua de Florida, and forcefully blow trago on his altar on the other side of the room, in preparation for the next ceremony. He handed my friend Ariel a long white candle to rub over his body for the diagnostic reading, and then he sat down, palms up on his knees, and started to chant, calling his spirits helpers for help.

What did he do to me? I wondered. Where did this vision come from? How does this ceremony work and why? What does he know about how the world works that we don't? It made no sense to me that simply using candles and eggs and chanting could produce such profound results. I desperately wanted to know how this healing worked. I knew that the man with this ancient primitive ceremony had touched my heart deeply in a way no other Western teaching had before. Was this what I was yearning for?

MEETING MARGARET: A PAST LIFE

We packed our belongings and headed out of Don José's house. "Where do you want to go now?" Juan Carlos asked. All four of us were in a daze after the ceremonies with Don José.

"Maybe we should go have lunch somewhere and then go and visit another shaman," Ariel suggested. "Another shaman?" I protested. "I don't know if I can take it."

Samuel and Joyce, our other two companions, agreed with Ariel and so we went. Juan Carlos unraveled the list of shamans from his pocket and we decided to visit Don Esteban Tamayo and his two sons in the neighboring village of Karabuela. And there I had another experience with the supernatural power of the Andes shamanic healing ceremony that would change my life again.

I don't know how it happened or what triggered it. I have no idea how long it lasted. I had no possible logical explanation for it, even though I tried hard, for years, to understand it. I had a spontaneous glimpse of another lifetime. The vision was so vivid, so accurate and detailed, to the last button of my white dress, my white bonnet, and the black horses that pulled the ambulance that took my lifeless body to the hospital.

My name then was Margaret. I was born in the 1890s and lived in a highly respected section of Vienna, Austria. I was tall, slim, and about thirty-five years old. I suffered from severe depression. My family sent me to a mental institution, a sanatorium called Purkersdorf. One bright day I was released and taken back home. I arrived, in a panic, and threw myself from the top floor window of my family's house, killing myself instantly.

Deeply startled and shaken at the end of the ceremony, I had to go outside of the shaman's home and walked down the hill to the cornfields below. When I started to climb back up the hill, I became even more startled. To my amazement I recognized where I was from a dream I had had just a few weeks earlier, where I saw myself walking up that dirt road toward a white building, which I knew in the dream belonged to a shaman. It was the same white house. My whole sense of reality was challenged again, leaving me even more confused. Am I the reincarnation of that young woman Margaret? I mulled it over in my mind. Until then I used to make fun of people who said that they experienced past lives. But was it real? Did I make it up? I could not decide.

Two years later, I was assisting the South American shamans at the Dream Change Coalition's shamanic gathering at the Omega Institute. At the prodding of my friend Ariel, I told a group of participants my Margaret story. From the darkness of that night I heard a woman's voice say, "Hey, I'm from Vienna. I know the place." I was dumbfounded. As an official skeptic I had to go to Austria and find out, and I did. Almost ten years later I walked into the Wien Museum on the famous Karlsplatz and with the help of a student of mine who worked there, I found the evidence and made photocopies. You can imagine how I felt when I realized that my vision was not an illusion.

I realized that this past life experience was the source of my fear of heights, which I have suffered since early childhood. I also remembered that as a very young child I had this feeling that I did not belong here and constantly asked why I was here and what I was doing. After I experienced the vision, my fear of heights subsided dramatically; I no longer get the sweaty palms, the palpitating heart, and the heavy cementlike legs I used to have while looking down from a high window or roof.

A week after that experience in the Amazonian's Shuar Territory in Ecuador, as I was crossing a hanging bridge over a small but deep river, I stood in the middle of the bridge and started dancing in elation.

Later, as I stood on the top of a hill overlooking the sacred Valley of the Dawn, surrounded by the powerful volcanic mountains of Imbabura, Cotacachi, and Mojanda, many questions filled my mind. Did the healing ceremony with Don Esteban Tamayo trigger me to relive that experience and heal it? What state of consciousness was produced that enabled me to see it? Could standing barefoot on a muddy floor in a semidark healing room, wearing only my underwear and surrounded by the musty smell of cow manure, sprayed over with trago, and blown over by fire and tobacco smoke bring me back to this past life experience? Did it happen because I was holding a *chonta,* or Brazilwood, spear on my shoulders as Jorge was thrashing my head and bare body with a bunch of dry leaves, chanting an old Quechua prayer, and rubbing my body with fresh eggs? Or maybe the red and white carnation flowers did it? What are the secret powers these humble, uneducated (in the Western sense) people who have so little have that we don't? I desperately wanted to understand.

Upon returning home with the gifts of necklaces, spears, and musical instruments, I knew my world had changed, and I entered into eight months of a life reconfiguration process, which felt more like deep depression.

MAKUNAIMAN: THE MAN WHO MAKES OTHER PEOPLE'S DREAMS COME TRUE

Upon my return from my first Ecuadorian trip, I participated in a series of classes at the New York Open Center with Nan Moss and David Corban. I, along with some of the participants from those classes, cofounded the New York Shamanic Circle, a nonprofit organization that promotes shamanic teachings together with our own monthly events, including workshops with guest shamans from around the world.

The Shamanic Gathering at the Omega Institute, in fall 1998, is where I met my other great influence, Ipupiara Makunaiman (Bernardo Peixoto, Ph.D.), a Brazilian *pajé* (shaman) from the Uru-e-wau-wau (People of the Stars) tribe of the North Brazilian Amazon and his Peruvian *curandera* (healer) wife. The Uru-e-wau-wau tribe believe that they were sent to the Amazon from the Pleiades star clusters with an explicit mission to teach humans how to be guardians of Earth. They knew that we didn't know how to live in harmony with nature and that Earth could be destroyed.

Ipupiara and his wife became my second most important teachers and mentors. I had the honor of assisting them in their many healings and trips. During a trip to Tuscany, Italy, to teach together, Ipupiara shared with me his life story. His introduction to shamanic healing was, as is sometimes common to shamanic practitioners, through shamanic sickness, death, and rebirth.

"I was born to a Portuguese man and a native Uru-e-wau-wau mother. At that time in 1933, we were only 2,400 people. I spent my early years in a small town in the rain forest, where my parents lived. My macho military father insisted that I become a military man like him or a priest: the two most respectable professions for men. My only brother did become a priest. In my early teens, I was sent away to have regular education in the city. It was a very difficult time for me: I missed my mother and the life at home. The children at the school in the city were so different from me. I was ashamed that my mother was a simple indigenous woman." His eyes teared up and he rubbed them under his heavy glasses.

"When I was about eighteen I got violently sick. The doctors in the local hospital could not figure out my sickness, and as I withered away, they gave up on me. They called my parents to tell them that there was nothing more they could do. My mother in her great despair begged them and my father to allow her to bring me back to her ancestral village. Delirious, I did not want to go there. I screamed at her not to take me back there. I was sure the shamans in the village would kill me. But she stood her ground fierce and stubborn like a mama jaguar. Despite my furious protests, she took me away, and we embarked on a two-day journey by car and by boat."

He stopped, put his two hands on his knees, and bent closer to me. He looked deep in my eyes and shook his head from side to side, letting his ponytail fly. "Would you believe that in two days the village shaman along with other healers cured me? They saved my life with herbal teas, bad-tasting herbal mud cakes, and baths, with other shamanic work done by our shaman. I slowly gained weight and fully recovered. Imagine, two days!"

He sat up and crossed his arms over his chest, smirking proudly. "I spent the next year in my mother's village, learning from her and other elders the ways of native healing. Then I had to go back to the university. I got a Ph.D. in anthropology and biology. After I moved to the

United States, I worked as a consultant at the Smithsonian Institution's National Zoo in Washington, D.C., and was an adviser to the White House. But what saddened me was that I was never allowed to go back to my mother's village." He started weeping again. "Why?" I asked. "For fear that I will infect them with the white man's diseases because I was away for too long," he said brokenhearted.

Ipupiara spoke eight local dialects, Portuguese, Spanish, English, and a little Italian. He and John Perkins cofounded Dream Change Coalition. I traveled with Ipupiara and his wife many times to their land in the Rio Negro in the Brazilian Amazon, where we met and learned from different tribes such as the Tukanos, Baré, and Ipixoto. At the time of his passing on May 16, 2011, there were only a handful of Uru-e-wau-wau alive. He was their last shaman. He has now returned to his waiting family in the Pleiades.

EAGLE BAPTISM

It was on my second visit to Don José eighteen months later in 1998 when I started to get some answers. A new mesmerizing vision that I had at his home prompted him to ask me to come back and become his apprentice. But not before he publicly reprimanded me for not following through with the bath instructions he had given me eighteen months before. How did he know that? I guess he sees everything, I thought to myself.

Once again I was standing almost naked in the middle of the room, my feet on an old newspaper with Audrey Hepburn's face, my favorite movie star. As the now familiar ceremony began, I found my body experiencing a total shape-shifting. At first I was afraid to let go and let it happen. Soon I realized I was turning into a full-blown eagle. Feathers sprouted on my entire body and hands. With the wide wings I grew, I powerfully thrust my body into the blue skies. At one point high above Earth I descended at huge speed deep into a small blue lake on a volcanic mountain. Then, as if by an unknown magical force, I flapped my wings and bolted up into the heavens, spewing the skies with tiny sparkling water drops like colorful shining diamonds. Again I could not tell what prompted this strange vision and how long it lasted.

When I heard our guide, Juan Gabriel, say, "You can dress now," I slowly opened my eyes. Audrey Hepburn was still there with her almond eyes smiling at me mysteriously from below. I was cold, exhausted, and shaken by the experience. Don José prescribed me a few things to do when I got home, including a few more flower baths, using red and white carnations and roses.

In our conversation later, I described my vision to Don José. "Oh, *claro,* that is the lake I take my apprentices for their initiations," he said seriously, shaking his head from side to side. He explained that I had had a baptism or initiation ceremony reserved for his pupils in a lake called Eagle Lake on Imbabura. I was stunned. What does that mean? How was I able to see his world? I doubted myself again. "Would you take me to this place one day in this reality?" I sheepishly asked him. "Oh, claro, no *problema,*" he said, smiling, his eyes glowing with mischief. He asked, "So, when are you coming back?" I promised him within a year, but my apprenticeship actually started in New York a few months later.

A WAR DANCE IN TARUMA

It was yet another hot and muggy day in the Brazilian Amazon. Shoré the Kanamari pajé was pacing in large circles in the center of the open-sided thatched-roof hut. His eyes were half closed in deep concentration; in his right hand he held a Brazilwood spear as he began the unfamiliar ceremony. I had come to Taruma Eco Center with eleven other North Americans guided by my mentor and teacher Ipupiara and his wife. They had built this center and school on the banks of a lagoon, near a tributary of Rio Negro, on what once had been an old boatyard. They wanted to transform its oily soil back into fertile ground.

I admired Shoré's decorated tribal clothing; he wore a large colorful macaw feather headpiece, his old face painted with the black markings of a jaguar. His bare upper body was adorned by many necklaces with different color seeds and alligator and wild boar teeth. His bare feet were strong as they pounded the mud floor. He is as real as it gets, I thought. Standing on the side were his wife, his daughter Daka, a powerful shaman herself, her two young children, and Aristeó, his younger apprentice from the Sateremaue tribe, all with painted faces and dressed in ceremonial clothing as well.

I was very tired and supercharged, as the night before, around three in the morning, I had woken up with a jolt. Sleeping lightly, I heard some unexpected sounds. From my hammock, five feet away from the thick jungle, I had a strange feeling a jaguar had just passed by me. Was it a dream? I wondered. The moon was full and bright, and I peeked out through the mosquito net trembling with gut-wrenching fear. I dared not move, waiting for the sun to come up. Finally, two hours later, I climbed down from my hammock and carefully walked to the place where I had heard the sounds coming from. There, close to the path that led into the jungle, I saw jaguar footprints, electric eel bones, and fresh poop. I held my breath and thanked God it wasn't my bones.

Ipupiara, my mentor and teacher, translated Shoré's words from Kanamari, his native dialect. "Come to the center," Shoré said, pointing at me. I stood up from the wooden bench and joined him. He then signaled three other men from our group to come to the center. We stood there not knowing what to expect.

Earlier, when he introduced him, Ipupiara had explained that Shoré is not his real name; in the Kanamari language it means "best man" or "best shaman." He said that Shoré received this name from other elders in recognition for his vast knowledge and the power of his healing. His tribe is located in the area close to Venezuela's border, so it took him and his family three days, by boat, bus, and another boat, to arrive at Taruma Eco Center.

Shoré took a few steps and pulled a stash of four red Pau-Brasil or Brazilwood (*Caesalpina echinata*) spears from under one of the benches. This rare dense wood, which Brazil is named after, is used for making warfare implements and other tools in place of metal. By Brazilian law, it is not allowed to be freshly cut, and only natives can gather fallen branches for making tools.

We stood in line facing him, and he handed one spear to each of us. He was talking as Ipupiara translated. "I choose to initiate you and gift you part of my personal power. I recognize that you have special power and commitment," he said. "But before I bless you, you each need to pass a test." He then asked the other three to sit down on a bench. I stood alone in the center, confused, aware of the many watching eyes. What is he going to do to me? I wondered. I could feel butterflies stirring in my stomach. What if I fail the test in front of all these people who know me so well? Maybe I'm not worth his trust. Maybe I'm not a powerful enough warrior to hold that sacred spear.

I was deep in my self-doubts when Shoré, a short old man in his seventies, faced me and fiercely struck the spear in my hands. Somehow that blow triggered an energy surge; it shook me to the core of my being, like I was struck by lightning, and by instinct I attacked him back forcefully without mercy. He struck me back from a different angle, and then from above the head and then below at my legs with surprising agility and force. I found myself grounding my feet in the pressed clay floor in a battle for life and death, not just protecting myself but also smacking him back. My heart was beating fast, and I noticed that although he was smiling his breath became heavier. We engaged in a forceful dance of war and wills for many long minutes.

Suddenly it was all over. We stood facing each other, breathing heavily. He looked me in the eyes and smiled with approval. I guessed I had passed the test. I bowed to him, thanked him, and went back to sit on the bench, holding my new spear tightly and catching my breath. What just happened? I asked myself. Where did this wild uncompromising warrior energy in me come from? At that moment I was so thankful to my son for taking me to kung fu classes many years ago.

At last, when the other three ceremonies were completed, Shoré invited everyone, including his family, to stand in line behind each other. He took his place at the head of the line and with small steps we began the traditional ceremonial anaconda dance to welcome the four new initiates.

"Think of me whenever you use this spear, and I will help you in spirit," Shoré told me, just as he was leaving on his journey back to his village. I thanked and hugged him strongly. I do so quite frequently, as part of him is in me forever.

THE RELUCTANT SHAMAN

It never crossed my mind that one day I would be chosen by a real indigenous shaman to become his apprentice. I also never dreamed of becoming a healer or even thought that I had what it takes to become one. Throughout the years, with a bit of skepticism but curious to know my future, I would go see psychic readers, card readers, and astrologers. I was fascinated and admired the uncanny abilities of those spiritual-ists, and I was curious to know their secrets. Aneeahseah Lefler, a great energy healer I met many years ago, told me that she saw me traveling all over the world doing healing and teaching shamanism, which I do now. But back then it shocked me to no end. I had read Carlos Castaneda's and Lynn Andrew's books, and I assumed an apprenticeship only hap-pens to special people, surely not an ordinary person like myself.

A year after my second healing with Don José, he arrived in New York to visit his family. We met for dinner, and on our way to a Chinese restaurant he stopped abruptly on a busy street in Queens. As a flicker-ing neon light shone on us, he turned to me, looked straight into my eyes, and asked with a strong voice, "Did you start to do healing?" I laughed and looked at him in disbelief. I asked Natalie, my translator, to confirm what he just said. "Who, me? I don't know anything, and I am not a healer," I protested. "Yes, you are, and you are ready; you should do it. Start now," he said seriously and demandingly. I was con-fused and did not know what to say. "What is it that I got myself into? Is he really pulling my legs? What does he sees in me?" I thought to myself. "If you think that I can do it then maybe you can teach me everything you know," I said to him, somewhat taken aback.

A few weeks later, I invited some of my friends to have healing ceremonies with him in my advertising agency's office. As Don José performed them, I sat there unsure of what my role was. He never said a word. He let me figure it out by myself. He really never taught or explained what he was doing and why it was customary in his culture. I tried to observe and memorize how he set up his altar. I listened to his chants and tried to remember when to light him a cigarette, how to shake the eggs on clients' bodies, how to blow the trago and Agua de Florida, and so on. Every time I had a question, he brushed me off. "Just concentrate," he demanded. I learned not to ask questions. There were no books or instruction manuals to read. There is no university or institution that teaches this, and you definitely can't take notes in the middle of a session. There were only lunches or some free time in the office when he let loose and told me things. He would share with me, through the translation of his English-speaking daughter, some stories and anecdotes of his life and healing incidents. Through these stories I was able to fill in the gaps of information.

One Saturday morning, as I watched him intently from my chair behind the altar, in the middle of a La Limpia ceremony, Don José whispered to me to take his place and carry out the egg clearing. I was shocked. "Me? Are you sure?" I looked at him. "Claro," he motioned me with his head, "come quickly." I suddenly felt nervous, my stomach queasy. I got up from my chair, took the two brown eggs from his hands, and started shaking them over the client's body, just as I saw him do so many times before. I was relieved the client had her eyes closed. She may not notice it's not him, I thought to myself. He seemed pleased and went on to finish the ceremony.

Over time, he would, always unexpectedly, motion me to do different parts of the ceremony, while closely observing me with his sharp critical eyes. Witnessing the immediate impact the ceremonies had on our clients, I was truly excited. I wanted more people to know of his work. I invited him to give a few workshops to my New York Shamanic Circle and for other interested people in New York.

Being an apprentice was not easy, and maybe it should not have been. Don José, only few years older than me, treated me like the son he never had. We became family. With tough love and high expectations, he demanded total loyalty. But I was naturally a curious person and had chosen to live in New York City because it is a pluralistic and open society. I celebrated different points of views and wanted to learn from shamans from other traditions too. Don José could not understand or accept my desire to do this. "I teach you everything you need to know from my tradition. Why go to someone else?" he scolded me in dismay. Our relationship went from hot to cold to hot to cold over the nearly sixteen years I studied with him. It was difficult to bridge our two worldviews, along with the language barrier and differing cultural expectations, but despite our differences, I absolutely love him and admire his vast knowledge and expertise.

THE FRUIT SALAD APPROACH

Ipupiara, my other teacher, somewhat sarcastically called the mixing of different traditions "the fruit salad approach." By taking something from each tradition and mixing it up, you can't taste each individual fruit independently. He mocked the enthusiastic students who had just discovered shamanism and were already trying to improve on it by mixing many traditions and disciplines together. He told me a story of holding a medicine bundle workshop in a midwestern city when a previous student of his ran in and said with excitement, "Ipu, Ipu, I want to show you my new medicine bundle. You will be so proud of me."

"Sure, why not, show it to me," Ipu said to her. "Oh, no," the student said, "I need to show it to the whole group, and I need to turn the lights off. The room must be in total darkness." If there was one thing Ipu could not control, it was his ample curiosity. So he agreed.

A traditional medicine bundle is constructed of a special fabric or leather. Wrapped in it are an assortment of sacred power objects that represent the shaman's inner power and healing intentions. It could contain different grains, metals, minerals, feathers, animal bones and teeth, stones, and other objects important to the shaman. It is considered one of the most sacred objects that shamans use for healing and for protection.

So Ipupiara gathered the group, explaining that one of the students from a previous workshop two years ago wanted to show the medicine bundle she had made. They all sat quietly in a circle as the lights were turned off. With great anticipation Ipu waited to see the mysterious magical bundle.

"Itzhak, you would not believe what I saw," Ipu told me. "To my disbelief, from a package at the center of the dark room by the altar came flickering lights. Green, red, yellow, and blue, blinking fast like a Christmas tree, like that—ta, ta, ta, ta, ta—one after the other. When the light show was over, the lights were turned back on, and she came over and asked me, 'Ipu, isn't it amazing?' while the students clapped enthusiastically, like it was a Fourth of July firework. 'Ipu, you can't imagine how impressive it is when I use it in my healings. My clients love it,' she told me. She was waiting for my approval. Itzhak, what could I tell her?" Ipu sighed and took a big breath. "Once you teach the sacred, you have no control over how people interpret it. They want to sprinkle some modern magic powder on the old teachings."

When I worked with Ipu, I would often witness people like her coming up enthusiastically to him to tell him about a new healing system they were learning or inventing. He would always listen politely, and then later turn to me and whisper in my ear, "Same thing in different clothing."

Yes, we all want to move on, change with the times, and use the latest terms and discoveries that are hot or cool, such as quantum physics, nanotechnology, DNA activation, theta waves, and so on. Some people take many different methods after they have studied them for a short while and mix them up to create a new method and then give the new method a fancy name or, worse, call it by their own name. For traditional shamans, Mother Earth is doing the healing, and the ancient way is sacred and needs to be honored. Nevertheless, having lived in the United States for a while, Ipupiara learned to understand and accept our lunatic frame of mind.

Don José's resistance to my wanting to learn a variety of techniques is not unique. I have heard of similar situations from others who became apprentices to indigenous shamans. We struggled to bridge our two different cultures, with our different expectations and cultural codes of ethics. Frictions are bound to happen. But on the other hand how else can we learn from one another?

THE CANDLE-READING DISCOVERY

For two years I sat behind Don José's back as he read the diagnostic candle flames at the beginning of the ceremony. Each time I was surprised at how accurate he was. I was determined to figure out how he did it. For two years I asked him to teach me or even just to drop me a small hint so I could learn it. "Concentrate," he continued to demand. Surprisingly, one Saturday morning it happened.

As he read for a heavy-set middle-aged woman, I looked from behind his back, as I always did, and lo and behold, I saw a dark blob in her stomach. I was so excited; I just knew I had figured it out. "She has a big problem in her stomach, maybe a big fear too," I whispered in his ear. "Shush," he said harshly and turned his head away, but not before I saw that mischievous sparkle of approval in his eyes. I had a great feeling of elation.

Today, I teach this diagnostic technique throughout the world, with additional information from my Brazilian mentor Ipupiara, in much less time than it took me to learn it. I am excited that many Western shamans are incorporating this technique in their regular practice.

BECOMING A YACHAK

In the spring of 2000, with my family by my side, Don José initiated and crowned me into the Circle of 24 Yachaks. First, ceremony was held under the moonless cold night sky at the foot of Imbabura, the formidable volcanic mountain, at the icy cold waters of Magdalena Spring, which feeds Imbakucha (La Laguna de San Pablo). A day later ceremony continued at Don José's home in Otavalo with a special ceremony, just us, with no one else in the room, using the chonta spears. I was not anticipating or requesting to be initiated; it did not even cross my mind. It was his decision. I felt tremendous gratitude and honor for being recognized, but at the same time my heart was heavy with the immense responsibility of carrying such old family tradition on my shoulders and being worthy of it. I still have the same feelings before each session I do.

It is not uncommon that many shamans are kept in the dark after a healing session, not knowing the short- or long-term effect of their work. Although common sense says that shamans do not need to be validated or live by the results of the healing they performed, on a human level, it is empowering and rewarding to know. I have many stories of clients that come years later, telling me how grateful they are and how the session we had changed their lives. It is always nice to know. What follows is the story of a woman I helped heal, which made a lasting impact on me.

SHARON'S LAST WORD

Sharon, a woman in her late fifties from Princeton, New Jersey, called me. "I'm calling you because I read an article written about you in *Breathe* magazine. I was diagnosed with cancer. I have already gone through the traditional chemotherapy procedures, but I know it's not enough. I want to heal and to feel better again." She spoke in a whisper, as she was very weak and desperate after her chemo treatments. Her loyal, big, and burly husband drove her in one Sunday afternoon, led her fragile body into my office, and patiently waited in their parked car. She came to see me every two weeks. After a number of months she regained her strength and became vigorous again. Her hair grew back. With her newfound enthusiasm, she began dreaming of her future and organizing a healing group and workshops for me in her house. She also started to study healing and had a busy social life. Too busy to come see me.

Three years later I got a phone call from a friend of Sharon's, who later became my client: "I'm sorry to tell you that Sharon's cancer returned. Her condition is worsening dramatically." I wanted to go visit her, but the following week I got a call that she had passed away. I was stunned. You can imagine how awful and disappointed I felt in my skills: I had not cured and saved her. I was so sorry that her college-age son and retired husband had lost her.

That same day I got a call from her family. They asked me to be present at her funeral. It was a sad and long train ride. The stone church was full of mourners when I arrived. Her husband greeted me warmly and led me to the open casket. I was startled. Sharon, with full makeup, lay there elegantly dressed and peaceful, covered by her favorite flowers. To my utter amazement I could not believe what I saw lying at her feet: a copy of *Breathe* magazine opened to the page containing my article. Tears started flowing freely from my eyes. Her husband, who saw my reaction, said quietly, "Yes, Sharon asked me to put it there as she knew she was going to pass on. She was so grateful that you gave her three more beautiful years." I hold her memory in my heart.

NOT JUST A SPIRITUAL BEING

Are shamans aliens who come from other stars, possessing superpowers? Are they rare enlightened superbeings, something like a guru? Many, including myself at the beginning of my journey, viewed shamans with a special awe, fear, and wonderment. The perception of a shaman as an enlightened being, a person who floats above our simple everyday life needs and tribulations with a permanent broad smile on his or her face, cannot be real. Shamans are simple human beings with a range of human feelings, desires, shadows, and virtues. They are just like you and me and should be allowed to be.

Perceiving shamans as special powerful beings is dangerous to anyone seeking help and to the community at large. A client might give away his power and thrust it in the shaman's hands. The client might hope that the shaman will puff a magic starry power on her and all will turn out fine—instead of the client being an active responsible participant in the process of healing. When you put someone on a pedestal, and he doesn't perform the way you imagine, it's easy to be disappointed and to knock him off. I learned this the hard way, of course, as it is hard to give up an illusion.

Many of the indigenous shamans I know have big open hearts and generous and loving spirits, and at the same time they also possess down-to-earth human vices. They can be proud, egocentric, passionate, righteous, possessive, and greedy and have a great need for power. To deal with the spirit world, you need to be a strong warrior, a powerful negotiator, and completely practical. There is no place for the faint of heart there. You have to make quick decisions as sometimes you or your clients are in a life-and-death situation.

Some shamans can be very competitive with one another; they up the ante against their colleagues, like a shaman I visited in Ecuador. I came to Ecuador with a group, and the shaman learned that a sick person from my group had earlier visited another well-known shaman. He belittled the other by proudly declaring, "Of course he could not heal you completely: he uses the energy and power of two mountains. I use those of three mountains." His surrounding family nodded in full agreement.

HOW MANY KINDS OF SHAMANS?

Two weeks before my wife and I flew to Santiago, Chile, to visit our daughter who was studying there, I had a strange dream early in the morning. An old man in his midseventies, with a head full of gray hair, intense black eyes, and bushy eyebrows, apparently a shaman, appeared. He said his name was Manuel.* "I am waiting to see you," he said. "But how can I find you?" I hastily asked him as he vanished into the thin air. I woke up and decided to follow up on that strange dream. I called my daughter in Santiago and asked her to help me find him. She made some inquiries, and people told her that a *machi* (shaman) is usually

---

*Note that I have changed his name here for privacy and protection.

a women's profession only; they dismissed my dream and suggested I make an appointment with a well-known woman shaman, not far away in the south, which she did for me. As it so happens, while we were visiting, my daughter shared with a taxi driver that I would like to meet a shaman and that we were on our way to Pucón in Patagonia. The driver laughed. "I am a Mapucé," he said. "And if you are going to Pucón, you must see Don Manuel; he is a very well-known shaman." My daughter was shocked. "But how are we going to find him there?" she asked. "Well, just ask. Everyone knows him," he replied. We cancelled the appointment with the woman machi.

As fate would have it, I asked the first person I met at our *hostería* and he knew of Don Manuel. So, we easily found him in his humble wood frame home by a beautiful blue lake the next day. Don Manuel looked like the man in my dream. He explained that in his Mapucé tradition, and perhaps in other cultures as well, there are three types of machi, each specializing in a different area. There is the herbalist, who heals with plants and herbs, the bone setter, who is similar to a chiropractor, and the spiritual healer, who performs community ceremonies and rituals and is available for consultations to resolve emotional and life issues.

Sometimes one person, like Manuel, can cross over and do some or all three of these disciplines; for example, I witnessed him fixing a young man's broken shoulder. Each role is important, and there is no hierarchy as long as the shamans bring healing to their clients or their community.

BLACK AND WHITE SHAMANS

There are essentially two types of shamans: The benevolent white shaman works with high vibrational energies and spirits of light and love; his or her intention is to reinstate the flow of life energy, balance, and harmony. On the other side there is the black shaman who works with dark heavy energies with the intention to stop or slow life energy, induce imbalance, create chaos and conflicts, and inflict harm. In many cases the result can be illness or even death. In some societies shamans operate from both categories, depending on their clients' requests or payments or the shaman's conscience or lack of it. In some shamanic cultures, these different roles of a black or white shaman reflect the social stature of the shaman, and the color of the shaman's ceremonial outfit can identify what kind of shaman he or she is.

Don José, who treated many shamans who used black shamanism and who were, as a consequence, afflicted by various ills, warned me to "never deal with black shamans or do black shamanism. If you send negative energy toward any person, it will come back to hurt you." In many indigenous communities, threats to use the evil eye to settle a score are common. Many people use shamans to settle long quarrels or take revenge on their enemies. Some believe that all deaths are the consequence of negative human intervention. The temptation for the shaman can be great to help facilitate revenge in return for money, gifts, and power. I experienced this at my home in New York, as the following short story illustrates.

One hot August night I was asked to host a Tsáchila shaman from Santo Domingo de Los Tsáchilas Provine, Ecuador, for a ceremony in my home. This man, who had never ventured outside his community, much less the world outside Ecuador, was shocked by our culture. His community still lived pretty much in their ancient traditional ways in the western rain forest of Ecuador. The shaman, in his midthirties, wore a traditional short black-and-white decorated skirt, with the red paste of achiote fruits painted on his head and bare chest. He conducted a beautiful nighttime ceremony. At the end of the evening, he offered us a short ayahuasca ceremony. As the night progressed, this peaceful smiling shaman drank heavily of trago. Soon he was intoxicated with the mixture of ayahuasca and alcohol. He told more stories and at one point became angry and aggressive.

As the circle dispersed, he followed me around, put his hand on my shoulder, his face close to mine; he looked straight into my eyes and fiercely said in broken Spanish, "I'm strong; everyone is afraid of me. If you give me a hundred dollars, I'll kill your enemies." I looked at him in surprise—to say the least. I was not sure how to respond to his offer. I was afraid to reject his proposal and make him angrier, but I could not entertain the offer either. "Oh, it's really not necessary. I don't have enemies," I finally replied. He took his hand off me and staggered away, disappointed.

WHO CAN BECOME A SHAMAN?

All humans, I believe, have the natural ability to "see" visions and to heal others, and as a matter of fact without even being aware of it, we are practicing these gifts all the time. When we have visions in our dreams or daydreams, follow our intuitive gut feeling or knowing, have déjà vu or an out-of-body experience, or have a past life vision, we are practicing a kind of shamanism. We are healers when we smile at someone on the street, gently touch or warmly hug someone, pray with good intentions, use comforting words or a soothing song, or listen attentively to someone whose heart is broken or who is in desperate need.

Ipupiara used to tell the students in his workshops, "You are all shamans, every one of you!" He would point to each person in the circle to emphasize what he was saying. "Don't think that just because someone wears feathers on his head, has long hair, wears a strange poncho, and has a hard-to-pronounce name or accent that he is more powerful than you are."

Once at the New York Shamanic Gathering in Central Park, hosted by the New York Shamanic Circle on the large green meadow of the Great Hill under a beautiful blue autumn sky, Don José, wearing a colorful feather crown on his head, long black hair, and a blue llama wool poncho, asked the participants to choose a partner and face each other. Then he asked them to open their arms wide and give each other a long hug. After the giggling had subsided, he then proclaimed, "You are now all healers. You just engaged in an energy transfer for the purpose of healing." Remarkably simple, isn't it?

In a workshop I was teaching in a New York college, I asked the group of thirty students to close their eyes and raise their hands if the following questions pertained to them. "How many of you had a dream that came true?" Five people raised their hands. "How many of you had a feeling before the phone rang who was on the other end?" Sixteen people raised their hands. "How many of you had a déjà vu experience?" Ten people raised their hands. "How many people think they saw a spirit?" Eight people raised their hands. "How many of you have had an out-of-body experience" Three raised their hands. And so on. Experiencing spiritual phenomena is more common than we allow ourselves to believe.

We all have significant spiritual experiences at least once in our lives. We learn to call them weird, strange, or unexplainable. Most of us learned to hide it from our parents and peers for fear they would ridicule us or call us crazy. But the truth is that all of us are born with these abilities. Often I tell participants in my workshops that each of us is no more than a mobile phone. They look at me wide-eyed as I explain that like an iPhone we all have a physical body, which is our hardware, and a brain, which is the software, with a transmission center that enables us to receive and send messages. All we need to do is increase the signal bars on our "phones," increasing our receptivity. The fact that we do not see those messages coming in or going out does not mean they do not exist. How does the mobile phone know when to ring? Have you ever seen a message coming or going through thin air? We know that we are surrounded by billions of these messages at every second of the day in different frequencies. When we learn to acknowledge these qualities in ourselves and embrace them, it becomes easier to perceive ourselves as energy and spiritual beings—as shamans. A shaman must train his mind to perceive those messages; he is as powerful as the power of his antenna.

There are plenty of ways a person can become a shaman. In some traditional shamanic societies, that knowledge is passed on from father to son, mother to daughter, or grandparent to grandchild. Sometimes a child is chosen at birth to be a shaman because of a special birthmark, the way he came out of the womb, an additional finger, or other signs.

Some children are chosen after a near-death experience, through sickness or some other trauma. Some discover their power at a young age. Some in their midlife, like me. Some people hear the calling and act on it. Some resist it, and some are forced to take it. Not everyone needs to become a shaman or feels the calling to become one. There is no right or wrong way or better time to become a shaman. It's truly up to spirit to call on you.

However, not every person who takes a short lecture or long workshop on shamanism can put a plaque on his door. It takes a strong commitment, long training, experience, and, yes, time. It is not enough to know how to journey using a drum or perform healing ceremonies. To become a full-fledged shaman, one needs to use her skills for the benefit of her community at large, to become "the keeper of the fire." She has to be committed to the health, balance, and harmony of her community and the world. But what if people refuse to take it upon themselves?

The Story of Maria

Maria, a beautiful woman in her midforties, came once for a healing session. She was a beautician and was made up perfectly—with blond hair and impeccable makeup, wearing a beautiful white pearl necklace with matching earrings. As always in my first session I started with the candle reading divination to diagnose her condition. I took a look at the candle flame and immediately saw that she was a shaman; not only that but she came from a long tradition and that her father was a shaman in Peru. I was a bit confused. So I asked her if what I had seen was true. She looked puzzled. "Yes, it is true, my father was a very powerful and renowned shaman at home," she confirmed. I jokingly asked her to switch places with me. "Are you practicing it today?" I asked her. "No, no, I do not want to. I want a better life for myself," she answered, as she patted her blond hair. I looked at her in sadness and with a bit of envy. I wished I had her lineage.

I looked again at the candle flame and had a beautiful vision. I was transported to Machu Picchu, the ancient Peruvian city on top of the Andes. There sticking out of the edge of a stone wall that surrounded a house was a large carved gray stone with a large serpent head. I described it to her. She gasped. "It's our family emblem," she said with tears in her eyes. We sat quietly. I was speechless. Here sitting directly in front of me was an authentic shaman from many generations of shamans, and she was running away from her heritage to a hair salon on Staten Island; what a waste. I took a look at the seeing and healing lines on her palm, and sure enough, she had those lines too. I was debating with myself if I should tell her what Ipupiara often used to tell me about people who refused the call. And then I looked in her big brown eyes and just said, "You have to practice. You have been given a gift and a responsibility. If you don't use it, you will get sick, because that healing energy must find a way to be practiced."

She looked at me, taken aback. "I know, I know. My father always used to tell me that too." She lowered her eyes. As if to herself she said, in a low voice, "Maybe I will consider that now." We sat for a long minute in silence. After her La Limpia ceremony, I saw in her eyes that something had changed, that she had begun to accept who she really is.

I did not hear from her until two years later. "Do you remember me?" the Peruvian beautician from Staten Island asked me on the phone. "I saw you about two years ago?" "Of course I remember you," I answered. "I'd like to see you again, soon."

As we sat again around my altar, Maria was terribly depressed and fidgeted. "What is the problem?" I asked her. She slowly raised her eyes to meet mine and quietly said, "I just found out I have cancer." We sat in a long pause of quietness. "I'm so sorry to hear that," I finally told her. "No, I did not follow up on becoming a shaman or healer," she quietly responded.

MAKING A LIVING AS A SHAMAN

Don José once told me (other native shamans I know also agree with him) that he sees his gifts simply as work. Being a well-respected yachak is not his only work: he once had a felt hat factory; he works his land cultivating corn, beans, and herbs; he has kept tomate de árbol orchards; and he's even sold Ecuadorian artifacts in street fairs when he comes to New York. "It is important for any shaman or healer to also have another day job. It helps him to keep himself grounded and not to be disconnected from the real everyday life of the people who seek his advice and healing." I have followed his teaching. I still own a design and advertising agency in New York City although I find myself spending more and more time on my shamanic activities. Both my teachers— Don José and Ipupiara—never viewed themselves as "spiritual" teachers but rather as professionals who worked with spirit to effect useful changes on behalf of their clients and their community. They insist that shamanic healing must be practical and results oriented to be effective. A Native American saying puts it in another way: "Does it grow corn?" If it doesn't, it means nothing.

Still, even if a shaman supports himself in other ways, shamanic healing is work and needs to be compensated. Some people believe that all healing should be offered for free as a gift from spirit, because it comes from spirit in the spirit of *ayni*—the universal way of reciprocity. Some believe that it is up to the client to offer what he can afford in exchange. Others believe that a client should pay a sum that is just above her means to show respect for the healer and to indicate that she is invested in the healing. Some practitioners take a percentage of the yearly income growth of the client, as a way to participate in the abundance of the client's experience.

Some believe the client should pay an agreed-upon price for the time the shaman spends with her. Ipupiara believed in that. He used to say, "You do not pay me for the healing, as all healings are priceless; you can't pay me enough for that. What you are paying me for is my time."

No matter what point of view you choose, I believe that an equal energy exchange must occur between the client and the shaman; the client must give something back, even if it's just a feather, a stone, a poem, a painting, or a food item. This gift is necessary not just as a sign of appreciation but also as a way to equalize the energetic relationship between the shaman and his client. When someone gets something for free, he tends to be in debt to the healer, and that lessens him and makes him dependent. That dependency usually creates anger toward the shaman. When you enter into an exchange, you are both engaged as equal partners, and the client must take full responsibility for her own healing.

In our modern life a healer also must pay for rent, mortgage, food, and other life necessities. In traditional societies, clients came to the healers armed with the necessary healing ingredients like flowers, eggs, alcohol, and so on, and with gifts, including food. They showed appreciation for the invaluable services the shaman performed, and they believed that her and her family ought to live a respectable life. Today, we have a different energy exchange system called money. I do not know a single shaman that is doing his work because of money; there are no rich shamans as far as I know. But I have seen many shamans and healers who are destitute and struggling badly. They can't pay their rent and are amassing debts; they live in poverty, existing on handouts, just because they believe that healing should be a gift. I always ask myself how they can contribute to the well-being of others when they themselves are not doing well.

In the High Andes, to be a yachak is a job, just like a weaver, a hat maker, or a farmer. Would you not pay a doctor because he is curing you? Would you not pay a therapist because he or she is doing it from the heart? It is no different for a yachak, who is working with spirits to heal you.

There is no right or wrong when it comes to compensation and energy exchange. It is up to each individual practitioner to see what works for her.

AN INTUITIVE PRACTICE

In addition to Don José and Ipu, I have been fortunate to meet and study with other outstanding medicine men and women from many cultures: Inuit, Maya, Aztec, Brazilian, Native American, Sami, Mongol, Tungu, Siberian, and Maori, to name a few. I learned and experienced the work of Don Alberto Taxo, Don Jacho Castilio,

Don Esteban Tamayo and his two children, Dona Maria Juana and Don Antonio Yamberla, Don José Quimbo Pechimba, Don Oscar Santillo, Susana Tapia Leon, and some others. I received valuable shamanic nuggets from all of them, which I have respectfully incorporated into my work. Words cannot express my thanks to them.

I truly wish these amazing and knowledgeable elders could have written this book. I learned that they did not believe in writing books. Many times I had asked my two teachers to write down their teachings, thoughts, and healing techniques, and many times I got vague answers: "Maybe . . . one day."

There is a reason why it's hard to find a book written by indigenous shamans, prior to the last few years. The concept of writing down wisdom and teachings their ancestors or spirits verbally passed on to them, which they do not own and which they believe belong to everyone, is unthinkable. Shamans believe that knowledge should not be frozen in pages of books. Knowledge is a living thing; it changes every day like nature itself. There are only a few things that do not change: the place where the sun rises and sets, the seven directions, birth, and death. Writing healing knowledge and wisdom on a piece of paper and binding it between two covers cages their energy and does not allow the reader to develop and grow on his or her own. So, as you read these pages, I encourage you not to follow my words but to use your own intuition and experiences.

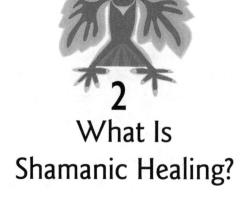

2
What Is
Shamanic Healing?

This is what today's world needs as an antidote to the greed of Homo economicus: *the wisdom of the indigenous world for collaboration, cooperation, mutual support, and respect for all of life. This is what the world's traditional, indigenous healers are providing people that conventional medicine is not.*

LEWIS MEHL-MADRONA, M.D., PH.D.

The millennia-old tradition of applying Earth-based techniques with vibrational energy and unseen spirits is generally called shamanic healing. These techniques include energy manipulation; use of sound vibrations, minerals, aromatic oils, and prayers; dietary advice; plant and herbal remedies; bodywork treatment; deciphering dreams; and work with the spirits of ancestors, entities, sacred objects, and nature through entering a trancelike state by consuming hallucinating plants, using sounds like drumming, rattling, or chanting, and performing rituals and ceremonies.

THE QUECHUA PEOPLE
AND THEIR HEALING SYSTEM

I was trained in the Quechua healing system as it performed in the village of Iluman by my teacher's family. The Quechua, or Kichwa, as they prefer to be called in Ecuador, are an indigenous ethnic group that reside in the province of Imbabura, which is named after the mighty dormant volcanic mountain that stands above the fertile, sacred Valley of the Dawn, and they are also in Colombia, Peru, Bolivia, Chile, and Argentina. The many ethnic groups that composed the powerful Incan empire, who called themselves "children of the sun," lived in these geographical areas and were united under one Quechua language. Even today there are more than eleven million Inca descendants, who may not all be pure blooded but who speak Quechua in many different dialects.

The Otavalan Quechua (Otavalo is their central capital), who live in the area my teacher, Don José, is from, maintained, against all odds, their traditional identity, with unique music, hairstyles, clothing, handicrafts, festivals and rituals, and belief system despite the Incan and Spanish conquerors and the strong influence of Western industrial high-tech society. Throughout the five hundred years the Spaniards ruled the Quechua, all healing and ritual practices were banned, and the Catholic religion was forced on them.

Despite this the yachaks continued to secretly perform their healing tradition, in hiding and under the cover of darkness. They started to come out in the open only in the late 1980s when their condor and eagle prophecies were revealed to the world. In 2008 the Ecuadorian constitution guaranteed the indigenous their rights to have their traditional medicine. Today there is an indigenous cultural revival: they have started to protect their sacred temples and *huacas* (sacred objects) and to be proud of their ancient knowledge and culture. Even health clinics and hospitals that incorporate shamanic and Western medicine together are now opening.

The Otavalan are known to be extremely hardworking, industrious, and practical people. They claim that they have had to be, since they were forced into hard labor to produce high quotas for the Spaniard colonialists and they lived in the harsh high-altitude weather of the Andes. This is why I also believe the healing system they developed is also highly practical and time tested.

The Quechua yachaks of the Otavalo area are the healers and spiritual leaders of their communities. They practice many forms of healing techniques. I have experienced some of them myself through Don José. Some, like my teacher, are still very traditional, and some who are younger and more "educated" infuse newer approaches into the old tradition. Some use sound healing and movement, and some stick to the old-fashioned ways in their practices.

Every yachak's family develops its own style and adaptations and sometimes, since the Inca had the practice of mixing ethnic populations throughout their empire, some shamans mix different traditions as well in their work. You can also sense a strong Christian Catholic influence incorporated into the prayers, altar, and visual presentation on their healing walls. But essentially they hold to a few core beliefs.

THE QUECHUA BELIEF SYSTEM

The Quechua revere the eternal living spirits of nature's forces such as the *apus* (mountain gods), Pachamama (Mother Earth), Taita Inti (Father Sun), Mama Killa (Grandmother Moon), Taita Waira (Father Wind), Mama Unu (Mother Water), Mama Ch'aska (Mother Star), and others. In their creation story, it is said that when Taita Inti chose to help humans after Jatun Pachakamak (Wiraqocha, Great Creator) created the universe, he made humans promise never to build or grow more than they needed, to become the guardians of Mother Earth, and to understand that they are connected to all things he created—the plants, animals, rivers, mountains, rocks, sky, and so on.

The Quechua and many shamanic indigenous traditions have three core beliefs: that everything that exists in the universe is alive and contains spirit or conscious energy; that the physical world, as we know and experience it through our five senses, is illusionary—it's nature and in constant change; and that the invisible worlds, which are composed of spiritual entities in the form of teachers, deities, ancestors, and so forth, are the only permanent worlds, and they interact and impact our daily lives, actions, and thought patterns. In addition the Quechua hold these basic beliefs:

- Jatun Pachakamak, the great creator, created everything in the universe perfectly and in full harmony, otherwise why would he do it.
- Because the universe is made of energy, healing can be done on an energy level in the seen and unseen worlds.
- Humans are one with the universe, and we are in relationship with everything around us.

The Quechua believe that the human body, like the universe, consists of two complementary parts: the physical body and the energy or illuminating body (also called *aura* or *parana*). This translucent illuminated body is an egg-shaped energy field that surrounds the physical body. It has two energy poles: a North Pole, a few inches above the head, that sends out positive ions and a South Pole, a few inches below the feet, that sends out negative ions. Each pole constantly sends energy beams, thus creating an electromagnetic shield that encapsulates our energy and keeps unwanted energy from penetrating us, much like Earth is protected by the energy shield of the atmosphere. In that energy field we store our memories, traumas, old spirits, and the energies of our ancestors.

According to the Quechua shamans, the human body can also be divided into four symbolic regions, represented by the four cardinal elements: earth, fire, water, and air. The head represents air (in Spanish, *aire*). It is the place of thoughts, ideas, visions, and intelligence. The pectoral area represents water (*agua*), the place of feelings and emotions. The midsection or groin represents the sacred fire (*mosoc-nina*), where passion, sexuality, the vitality of life-giving forces, and creativity are stored. Finally the legs, which represent our connection to Earth (Pachamama), indicate the way we stand in the world, how rooted and grounded we are.

Andes tradition believes in the reincarnation of the spirits of the dead or *ushai* (soul, spirit), which are believed to be released out of the body at the time of death. Ushai is the fifth element and is as important as the other four—earth, fire, water, and air—since it the union of all of them.

Don Alberto Taxo, a Cotopaxi yachak, teaches that the four psychic planes of soul, astral, physical, and mental are represented by the four elements of fire, air, earth, and water as well, which correspond to the four faculties within each of us, respectively passion, logic, material, and emotions. They represent different levels of vibration and frequency, which exist within the same space, like radio bands on which you can pick up different stations depending on their wavelength. Essentially they are protective casings that allow us simultaneously to experience life at these different levels. Since our consciousness is mostly held at the physical level, we need to make a conscious effort to communicate with the other planes to be fully authentic and engaged in our human experience.

IT'S ALL ABOUT ENERGY

Shamans believe, as science does, that the building blocks of all that exists in the universe are made of energy particles (atomic and subatomic), which, as they move in perpetual motion, rebound on each other, vibrating at different speeds and frequencies that create different physical structures. That vibrating energy is in essence what the shamans call consciousness or spirit.

Take for example the human body, which is made mostly of water, along with oxygen, carbon, hydrogen, nitrogen, and calcium and trace amounts of other elements. In addition, a few trillion of bacteria and viruses inhabit our bodies—comprising up to two pounds of our body weight. But that amalgamation of your cells with those bacteria and viruses does not make up who you are. What makes you uniquely you is the continuous eternal energy of your soul—which means there is no death. The essential elements of you don't die; they are transmuted. Ice, water, and steam provide a simple example of different states of being— the same element in different physical states. What makes these three states different is the speed at which the molecules are moving.

Our thoughts are the result of an electrochemical process. Specialized cells called neurons in the nervous system deliver messages from the brain to the body using electrical and chemical signals. Shamans believe that as they concentrate their intention and thoughts, they can transmit beams of invisible energy to the object of their healing. That enables them to interact with, communicate with, and influence the object and create a demonstrable change (As Japanese researcher Masaro Emoto demonstrated in his breakthrough experiment showing that intentional prayers affect the molecular structure of water). Shamans are also able to interact with other energies or the spirits of, for example, trees, stones, mountains, rivers, animals, and wind; they can learn from these spirits, communicate with them, and influence them. Shamans can send positive, high-frequency energy with messages or prayers for healing, or they can send negative, low-frequency energy to harm others. Quantum physics has come to similar conclusions, which is that the observer changes the outcome of the particles' behavior and that space and time is a construct of our consciousness.

THE SHAMANIC COSMOLOGY
AND HOW IT RELATES TO OUR HEALTH

Is the physical world we are living in the only one that exists? Are there any other invisible worlds? Are those who believe that "what you see is what you get" correct? Is only what is tangible and attainable by the five senses—touch, smell, taste, hearing, and seeing—real? What about those unexplained phenomena we have all experienced at least once in our lifetimes, such as foretelling future events, dreams that become real, visions or communication with the dead or other entities, and telepathy? How can we explain or prove their existence? Humans have asked these important questions since the dawn of civilization.

Many indigenous cultures believe that the known world, the physical world of the five senses, is only one of at least three. They divide the cosmos into three main portions: the lower world, the middle world, and the upper world. Shamanic cosmology was born out of humanity's profound observations of the natural forces and the mysterious phenomena of our world. It was created to help humans make sense, organize, and accept the inner and the outer worlds in which we live. For millennia, different cultures have developed similar observations, which have probably come from shared human experiences and needs.

The yachaks whom I studied with believe that this cosmological division can be seen in our own body as well. The legs represent the lower world, our connection to Earth; they are our roots. Strong legs are the conduits through which we bring the nutrients and fire into our furnace, or sexual organs. We must have strong legs to survive on this Earth.

The torso, the middle world, is the world of constant physiological and emotional changes. As a bridge between the lower and the upper parts, its digestive, respiratory, cardiovascular, and other systems need to be treated with care to keep them healthy and physically powerful.

The head, the upper world, is the place for thoughts, ideas, and spiritual practice and is our connection to the ethereal. We need to train this gate through meditation and prayer.

This cosmological division can also be viewed as the three stages of life: young age—the time of primary impulses, fertility, desires, and action; middle age—the time of change, of reasoning and questioning; and old age—the time of wisdom, reflection, and spirituality.

Each of these worlds contains different characteristics, symbols, powers, and consciousness. Each has a significant role, and each one is relevant to our physical, emotional, and spiritual life. These worlds are not, however, entirely divided; rather, there is a constant invisible energy flow among them through the center of Earth—or our body—and the six cardinal points. To see them and be able to work with them, a shaman enters a nonordinary reality, a shamanic state of consciousness.

The Lower World

The foundation of creation is the underworld or the lower world. It plays a big role in ancient mythologies such as the Egyptian, Greek, and Hebrew. Under the influence of Christianity, Hel, the Norse goddess of the underworld and the dead, was vilified and transformed and came to be associated with the concept of punishment by fire and the place where the devil and demons dwell.

Some cultures believe that there are a few levels to the underworld. Different shamans experience these differently in their trance visions. In some parts of Russia, shamans have identified thirteen levels. In the Mayan tradition there are nine, representing the nine levels of consciousness one needs to go through to reach enlightenment. In Norse mythology, there are also nine worlds, with the underworld ruled over by Hel. The ancient Hebrews believed that Sheol (the underworld) is divided into either four subsections or two major ones.

In shamanism the lower world is the realm that is associated with the mother, or feminine energy—the cycle of life, death, and rebirth. It is also associated with what is hiding, developing, and growing inside the womb. It corresponds to the element of fire, the transformative element that resides in Earth's core. Fire infuses us with our unique life force, our anima. It nurtures us and imbues us with primal passion and sexual potency. It's probably the reason why the male-dominated church was so afraid of the lower world and chose to vilify and subdue it.

It is in the lower world that the shaman connects to his animal spirit allies for the purpose of bringing messages and knowledge of healing for his clients.

The Middle World

The middle world is also called the physical or terrestrial realm. It is the material world in which we live and that we can easily grasp and interact with through our five senses; we can assess and measure it. We call it our normal world, our reality. Because of that, some of us consider it as the only existing realm.

In the shamanic tradition it is positioned between the two eternal worlds of heaven and the underworld. It is the world of continuous change and flow between two eternal worlds. Many old cultures see the sacred or world tree, with its roots deep in Earth and its crown in the sky, as representing the bridge connecting these two worlds.

In the shamanic tradition the middle world does not really exist. It is a world of dreams, illusions, and make-believe. "The world is as we dream it," as the shamans deep in the Amazon teach us. Why? you may ask. Because shamans believe that this world is formed solely by the movement of energy particles, which form the world we perceive and experience in our mind. More about that belief in the pages to come.

The middle world is represented by the element of water, which is symbolized by emotion—e-motion as energy in motion. The world is like water in that it is in constant change that, nonetheless, flows in one direction—from birth to death, from beginning to end. Water, the essential element for life, needs boundaries to contain it (the two other worlds), otherwise it is shapeless.

The middle world also possesses unseen earthly powers, magical forces, and spirits, as everything is alive and carries consciousness within it. Shamans journey to the middle world to connect with the spirits of mountains, springs, trees, stones, and other living or nonliving objects, to "see" or "visit" people or events in distant places, to bring knowledge, and to effect change in this realm.

The Upper World

In the upper world one can find the clouds, the air, the celestial bodies, such as the sun, moon, and stars—the entire cosmos. It's where the spirits of our ancestors, angels by many names, gods, and spiritual teachers of all traditions dwell. This is where the soul of the departed ascends to, and new souls descend through this world when they are ready to be materialized. Many spiritual cultures count more than one level in this world—seven, nine, thirteen, eighteen, and even ninety-nine. It is symbolized by the element of air. This realm represents thoughts, ideas, light, inspiration, and a broad perspective. Some believe that after passing through the lower world you emerge within this celestial realm, where we connect with the source of creation or God, Jatun Pachakamak. We think of it as heaven, a place of everlasting joy and bright light, contrary to the lower world, which is marked by death, sadness, and shadows. In Greek mythology Zeus, the king of the gods, rules that realm. Shamans journey to this world to obtain knowledge from the spirits of the ancestors and the dead. The upper world represents the masculine energy, the power of the mind, thoughts, and ideas.

THE PRINCIPLE OF BALANCE

At the core of the shamanic healing tradition is the belief that everything in the universe has two opposing yet complementary forces: dark and light, good and evil, the seen and unseen worlds, rainy and dry seasons, yin and yang. Both are needed to create harmony and balance. We all possess both feminine and masculine energies, the two opposing and complementary forces within us; this is not to be confused with one's gender or sexual orientation. In our everyday life we need both parts to be whole and to function with harmony.

The feminine energy center is in the left side of the body; it is the life energy that flows straight from the heart and is the source of our lifeblood. It's the ability to live with full trust, receiving with gratitude the abundance of the universe. It is the energy of walking in tenderness and beauty and the capacity to have faith and fully surrender. It is connected to fertility, motherhood, nurturing, compassion, and deep and turbulent emotions that can be transformed in an instant, much like the element of water. Like Grandmother Moon who shines on us in the dark of night by reflecting the bright sunlight on us, the feminine projects light on our hard-to-reach dark subconscious. This energy is associated with deep knowing, strong perception, and gut feeling or intuition. The feminine connects us to the womb deep inside Earth, life's core, giving forces that fuel creativity, fiery passion, and intense desires. It is the gravitational force that keeps us grounded to Earth and in reality.

Masculinity, on the other hand, is the energy of logic and thoughts, of big ideas. It is cold qualifying logic, calculated strategy, philosophy, and wisdom that comes from the ethereal world. It is practical and is removed from emotional energy and is symbolized by the blue sky. Its element is air, and without air there is no breath of life. Masculine energy expresses itself by taking a direct, aggressive, and active approach to life. It takes first and asks questions later. It is the warrior who is willing to strike, to kill and protect. Masculine energy is located on the right side of our body.

Honoring those two energetic forces the Quechua built great

temples that represented Taita Inti and Mama Killa. These two temples were built in every large population center on nearby opposing hills; some of them still exist but are no longer used for worshipping.

Some years ago, I visited the reconstructed temple of Templo del Sol near Pululahua Crater when the sun was at high noon. I entered the temple and walked for a few minutes through a dark circular tunnel, which signifies the birth canal a newborn passes through as he enters the world. I emerged into a high-ceilinged circular room flooded by bright white light that streamed through a small round opening at the cone-shaped apex of the ceiling. There were three rings of balconies all around the high walls, which were used by visitors for silent prayers and meditations. I watched a local young man walk into the white beam of light and was stunned when his body seemed to completely disappear in the powerful beam; the beam seemed to transform him into light. It's hard to describe my feelings and body sensations when I myself stood under that strong illuminating beam of light; it was as if the pure white sunlight energized and filled my batteries with healing transformative energy.

Unfortunately, many of the temples were destroyed or built over by the Catholic Church. The most famous one may be El Panecillo Hill in Quito. A huge and imposing statue, the Virgin of Quito, stands on the ruins of the ancient temple of the sun, looking down on the whole valley of Quito.

BALANCING THE
MASCULINE AND FEMININE

Unity and balance between the masculine and feminine parts are essential for any healing to occur. True healing must first acknowledge those forces and start an inner dialogue that can lead to honoring those aspects, a process that reunites them and brings them into a supportive relationship. That is why you will see on a shaman's altar objects that represent these two energies, such as red or white carnations or roses, eggs, musical instruments, and volcanic healing stones. During the healing ceremony, the shaman always begins the healing at the crown of the head and then moves to the left side (feminine) first, to open up the receiving energies, and then goes to the right side (masculine) to open the activation process. To be a good shaman one mustn't be shy to use the energies of both genders in one's healing practices as needed, even shape-shifting into the opposite gender.

To be healthy you need both energies or you become imbalanced, like a bodybuilder who overdevelops his upper body and neglects his legs, or people who develop their spirituality and forget their physical body. When someone has too much of one energy and too little of the other, the two forces clash with each other, which creates imbalanced behavior, builds tension, fosters conflicts at work and in personal relationships, and causes physical sickness. I'm sure you know men who are afraid to show their feminine side and so tend to be overly aggressive, or women who are afraid to show their masculine side and remain subordinate. The reverse is also true: men who are overly feminine and women who are overly masculine. A man or a woman who is too male is like a corporate lawyer who leaves his heart at home when he goes to work.

I have seen this imbalance in my practice many times.

ILLNESS THROUGH IMBALANCE

In contrast to Western medicine, traditional shamanic healing is not necessarily about curing someone's symptoms or manifestations of illness. Rather, it sees the sick person as a whole complex environment and makes an effort to reinstate the person's overall health. True healing happens by restoring harmonious balance and connection to nature and fostering oneness among the person's body, soul, and spirit. The shaman aspires to locate the deeper cause of the client's condition, which may be emotional or spiritual in nature, and bring the client back into alignment with his or her soul's calling, spirit's purpose, and daily path.

The Quechua strongly believe that all physical, mental, and spiritual problems are essentially the results of an imbalance in our energy bodies. This imbalance in our energy body results from polluted energy penetrating our illuminated body—that oval sphere that envelopes us.

Bad energy can be easily transferred through words and sounds, through our mind using curses and the evil eye, and through emotions such as jealousy and envy (*envidia*). If you become jealous or envious, for example, you can transmit that bad energy to your family, friends, and clients. Just being in or around physical places that contain negative air or wind energy (*mal aire* or *mal viento*), like the location of a murder, a battlefield, or a natural disaster can transmit negative energy to us. These conditions can occur by meeting harmful spirits (*duende*) or harmful energy attachments or intrusions sent either intentionally or unintentionally by another person as in witchcraft (*brujeria*). A trauma, shock, or sudden fright (*susto* or *espanto*) can unbalance the energy and cause a soul loss.

Negative energy (Supay) has a lower vibration. It is stagnant energy, thick, heavy, without life force, and essentially related to evil and death. Positive energy (Kawsay) flows freely, is moving and changing like life itself, and is recognized as light, a higher vibration.

The shaman's sole work is to bring his client back into a state of balance and harmony. An Ecuadorian shaman once told me, "Listen to me carefully. I'm going to tell you the three most important principles of shamanic healing: (1) be in balance with yourself, (2) be in balance with your family and community, (3) be in balance with Mother Earth. That's it. It is all about being in balance." Sounds so simple, but it is not.

This is the balance between the earthly heavy and dark forces and the heavenly forces of spiritual and light or the balance between feminine and masculine energies, found by opening all the energy blocks in the body. Opening the body's energy blocks and cleansing negativity will help to lift anxiety, depression, fatigue, and emotional trauma—opening pathways for happier relationships, peacefulness, better sleep, higher energy, better concentration, and the attainment of abundance.

Shamans believe that the major part of healing is done by none other than Mother Earth, herself, Pachamama. Mother Earth—who goes by other names: Alpa Mama, Mama Terra, Ima Adama—is the real healer. The shaman's body and spirit become a vessel that channels her energy and her vibrations, which do the actual healing. Therefore, the shaman must be humble and take no credit for the results of the healing he performs, as remarkable as the healing might be. As Ipupiara used to say, "Mother Earth is doing 50 percent of the work, the patient is doing 40 percent, and the shaman only 10 percent. So how can one take credit for that 10 percent?"

WHAT BLOCKS US

Many of us find ourselves asking the same nagging questions throughout our lives: Why can't I become a better and a happier person? What stops me from reaching my career goals or making money? Why am I so afraid of finding a partner or making a commitment in my relationships? Why do people always take advantage of me?

Sound familiar? We may feel helpless and not know what stops us from living to our full potential. Some of us take all the blame on ourselves: "I'm too weak, too stupid, too this, too that. I draw bad luck to me." Some blame others: "It's all my parents' or my siblings' faults. It's because of the place and circumstances into which I was born." Some feel they are the victims of an uncontrollable situation, and it is out of their hands: "I was in the wrong place at the wrong time." Likely, it's some of all of the above.

Energy blockages can be caused by a variety of incidents or circumstances. It could be a seemingly innocuous life event that is not easily remembered and has been brushed off as not a big deal. Or the client may have witnessed or experienced violence, a threat or trauma, or physical or sexual abuse. Many negative energy blockages originate from old fears, guilt, negative beliefs, and judgment put on us by our immediate family members. The blockage can also come from other people's curses, projected energetic hooks, or spirit attachments. Past life incidents or the unfinished business of ancestors and their interference in the client's life can also contribute to blockages.

These blockages are obstacles that get in the way of our material and spiritual abundance. Sometimes we feel we do not deserve to have what we want. We may have an inner wish to not take on responsibilities, as the more we have, the more we have to take care of.

DIAGNOSING
AND REMOVING BLOCKAGES

The shamanic healing way attempts first to find the true cause of the blockage or obstacle and then remove it from its root. Those blockages could be physical, emotional, or spiritual. By removing the obstacles that clog the river of life, it can flow freely again and restore the flow of the client's energy so she can become a more integral part of nature and society.

It is hard to see energy blocks and to locate them within you. We can only sense their existence in our physical bodies or energy fields using our intuition and sensory powers. Some shamans are able to see energy blocks as a dark mass in their clients' physical body or illuminated energy body. They learn to scan their clients' inner physical and energy bodies with their knowing eyes and intuitive feelings.

To diagnose blockages shamans employ a number of tools. They can connect with and receive information via their spirit helpers. Shamans in the Amazon and other cultures can see these blockages once they ingest special medicinal plants. Some can locate them through candle reading, in which a client brushes a candle over his or her body and the candle absorbs the client's energy. Once lit, the shaman can use it to spot any blockages. They may also read the reflections in obsidian and glass mirrors. Some shamans can lay hands on or above their clients' body and detect where negative energy lies by the different temperature it emits from the body. Some people can see it from far away. Some shamans see entities that intrude on a person's body in the form of people or animals. In my healing workshops, I teach people to successfully see and feel negative energies, and they are always surprised at their ability to do so.

Reinstating the energy flow clogged by those blockages can be a challenge. Throughout the ages, shamans have developed numerous tools and methods to remove these blockages and obstacles from their clients. Shamans can use ceremonies using the four elements: fire (transformation of the old), water (purifying and flow), air (blowing away), and earth (grounding). They make metaphysical incisions using metal or wood swords and spears, and they also use prayers and chants. Some use cord-cutting ceremonies to break a connection to an unhealthy relationship, deep breath work, and healing with sounds—all to remove those barriers. They can engage in soul retrieval, the process in which a shaman locates a missing part of the client's soul and reunites it with her client; shamanic journeys with spirit guides to seek knowledge and answers on behalf of the client; positive affirmations and meditations; fire ceremonies to burn old negative energy and bring transformation; curse removal; and much more. Of course, each culture or tradition does it differently and uses different ingredients based on its locations, but the principles are similar.

Throughout the healing session the shaman evokes the apus (mountain gods), the spirits of the four elements, and also the spirits of rocks, plants, rivers, and animals to awaken and activate the client's five senses: touch, smell, hearing, sight, and taste—and hopefully the sixth one by opening the third eye to "see." His goal is to infuse his client with feelings of emotional and physical well-being to induce balance and facilitate the process of healing. To accomplish this the shaman facilitates a deep connection between the patient and the feeling of oneness with the universe (the Great Creator). This is done through the opening of blocked energy channels among all four body areas and spirit.

Every item used in the healing ceremony is not chosen randomly by the shaman. Each item carries special spiritual energy and symbolic meaning and has been time-tested to bring good results.

In the following two sections, I explore in more detail healing with sound and working with nina, the sacred fire.

HEALING WITH SOUNDS AND MUSIC

Among the methods that Ipupiara taught was the drum-healing technique. He would say, "Sound vibration is like a deep tissue massage that penetrates the hard-to-get-to inner organs. It rearranges the physical and emotional bodies."

The shaman's voice and the musical instruments he plays have an important role in all shamanic healing traditions. Drums, flutes, rattles, ocarinas, bells, string instruments, and conch shells are some of the instruments that are used for clearing blocked energy, stimulating hard-to-reach inner organs, and cleansing the energy body that surrounds the physical body.

Some shamans incorporate sound into their regular sessions. They use it to first go inward to get into a trance and then outward to send their intentions to their clients. Some shamans use sound healing, which the Quechua call *taki sami,* as an exclusive method. They believe that the pulsation of musical tones interacts, rearranges, and activates the body's own vibrational energy. Sounds can invoke a state of ecstasy to bring about visions and heightened consciousness, can stir up negative energy and trauma trapped in the body's tissues and organs and thus enable them to flow out, or can harmonize the person with the vibrations of the universe or the Great Spirit.

The Quechua shamans believe that each organ in the body vibrates to different frequencies and the healer must harmonize with that frequency. The lower and heavy tones come from Earth, starting with the feet, while the highest tones come from above and aim above the crown of the head.

The composition of the instruments is of great importance; for example to heal knee and other joint problems, the shaman plays with reeds or bamboo flutes or panpipes because these plants have joints and grow in or near the water and so promote energy flow. Clay instruments, with their earthly lower tones, are best for the legs. Blowing the sounds of a conch shell, which suggests water, on a client's spine or other areas is good for emotional release. A high-pitched ocarina is used for the mind and higher consciousness. Metal bells or chimes in different tones are used for balancing both energy and the physical body.

I had a personal experience with the power of sound. It was in 1997 on my first trip to Miazal, a Shuar community in the heart of Amazonian

Ecuador during an ayahuasca ceremony led by the shaman Daniel Guachapa. He sat in front of me on a turtle-shaped wooden bench as I lay half naked on a bench made from a turned-over dugout canoe, which was set along the bamboo wall of the hut we were in. He opened with an icaro, or sacred spirit chant. The repetitive melody filled the thick, warm jungle night air. The vibrations of his raspy voice and the continued beating of the *chakapa*—a rattle made of dried leaves—filled my head and penetrated every cell of my body. I entered into a trancelike state and I let go. Strange visions started to appear in my mind, transporting me to different realities. His icaro guided his spirit helpers to release bad energy I had been accumulating for a long time. I found myself humming his icaro. "I passed on my teaching to you this way," he said the next day.

Don José chants and whistles throughout the entire healing ceremony. Doing this helps to transport his clients to altered realities, allowing them to relax their bodies so that healing can occur. "The voice vibrations are the gateway to connect to spirits," he said. He also uses a high-vibration bell and a high-pitched ocarina to connect the client with his or her soul.

Don Oscar Santillan, an Ecuadorian shaman, plays different flutes made of bamboo, clay, jade stone, and condor feathers and bones or the larger conch to stimulate the area of his clients that needs clearing and healing. Each pitch is directed to a different organ as the air or wind element moves and shifts inner body and out-of-the-body energies.

One bright and clear morning in Tumbaco, near Quito in Ecuador, I climbed a steep hill with Susana Tapia Leon and her client, an American musician and songwriter. Once we arrived at the top of the hill, she sat her client down on a rock facing the vast valley below and had her do some deep breathing techniques. She then instructed her to sing. At first the client produced lovely, childlike gentle sounds. "Go for more," Susana encouraged her. "I can't," she said, weeping. "I can't do it. I don't know how." Soon the woman started to cry hard. Susana let her discharge. "Now sing from your vagina, from your guts," Susana sternly instructed her. She sat behind her client, hugging her body strongly. "Start now," Susana demanded.

With a big effort first, the cracking sounds of a wounded animal came out of her open mouth. Childhood pain, unspoken grief, and deep-rooted anger were released into the void below. Susana kept embracing her strongly. "Now sing." This time a new voice came out of her client—clear, natural, and full. "I never let myself release those deep emotions before," she later confided to us as we made our way back down the mountain.

Waterfalls are an excellent place for sound healing in the same way. As you step under the gushing noisy water to clean your body, howl, scream, and pray to release the stuck energies in your body.

NINA: THE SACRED FIRE

According to Don Alberto Taxo, *mosoc-nina* means "sacred fire" in Quechua. The mosoc-nina energy center resides in the lower belly, about three fingers width below the navel. The nina enables us to be grounded and creates motion, strength, and balance. It is associated with the eternal flame, the life-giving force that radiates to the rest of our body and spirit. It is the furnace that empowers the rest of our body. It is the cauldron of passion and creativity and the womb where life is conceived and germinates. It is the source of sexual energy and vitality.

Other cultures also recognize that energy center in our bodies, and you may find different names and descriptions for it. In the Tree of Life of the Jewish kabbalah, it is Yesod, the foundation, the ninth Sefirah. It is called *dantien* in Qigong, *hara* in the Japanese tradition, or *kath* in the Sufi tradition. In the Hindu tradition of the seven chakras, it is the second sacral chakra, also called *svadhisthana*.

Nina is not about the sex drive; in fact, there is no word for sex in Quechua. Instead, the word describes the event when two people are engaged in the act of sharing sacred fire and in so doing merge the two most powerful male and female universal energy sources—the eternal fire of Taita Inti, father sun, and the passionate magma core of Pachamama.

Nina is the spark that resides in our body and soul. Awakening and restoring the sacred fire within my clients is an important part of my healing work. In my experience many people in our society for reasons of cultural conditioning and taboos, sexual abuse, trauma, and fears are unconsciously and consciously avoiding or hiding this part of themselves. It sits there like a dormant volcano waiting to explode, like a dam waiting to crack. If nina is blocked and not expressed, it can result in repressed anger and a life of resentment and depression, which can then lead to many afflictions and suffering. No wonder so many people in Western society are sedating themselves.

The shaman's role is to ignite that sacred fire, which then starts a chain reaction in the client's physical, emotional, and spiritual bodies. By pulling Earth's magma through the bare feet and up through the legs to the nina area, the connection between Mother Earth (earth element) and nina (fire element) is restored, and the client feels his or her power renewed. This life-giving energy starts to flow into our emotional body (water element), which includes the abdomen, lungs, and heart, and then goes through our throat, the place of expression, and on into our head-mind and thoughts (air element), which helps us connect to the heavens and spirit. Thus the flow of the river of light is opened, restoring the cycle of life and health and enabling us to connect to ushai, the fifth element, whose role is to unite and bring balance to all the elements of life. Don Alberto always said that it is important that the shaman himself intimately connects with, fully understands, and deeply feels the nature of each of the five elements in order to facilitate effective healing.

There are a couple of techniques for detecting the nina in a client's body. The shamans of the Andes use a candle-reading system, which will be detailed later on, but in short the client first rubs a white candle over his entire body and then the shaman lights the candle and examines the flame, in particular the area where the wick meets the wax. The color, intensity, size, and shape of the flame tells the shaman the state of the nina. Another technique is to place the palms of your hands over this area of the body and feel the temperature and energy that radiates from there.

LA LIMPIA: CEREMONIAL HEALING

The Andean traditional energy cleansing La Limpia is used frequently whenever people get sick, attract bad luck, or other misfortunes arise in their lives. It is a powerful physical and spiritual purification process that can balance the energy field by removing or extracting stale and negative energies. Many other shamanic traditions recognize the importance of clearing the illuminated energy field around us and have similar ceremonies using other means like feathers, smoke, crystals, water, and other methods.

La Limpia ceremony, like most shamanic ceremonies, is usually held at midday, midnight, sunrise, or sundown, as those are the most auspicious times of the day. These are betwixt and between times, when the borders of the physical and spiritual worlds blur, creating a portal through which a shaman and his client can enter into other worlds.

If this illuminated energy shield breaks down or becomes weak, outside negative energy can penetrate our energy field, and we start living in imbalance, which can then lead us to develop physical, emotional, and spiritual diseases. I'm sure you have experienced imbalanced energy penetrating your field; for example, while riding a subway or a bus, or being in a public place, you suddenly felt bad energy coming from the person sitting next to you or someone stared at you intensely and you started to feel bad yourself. Perhaps you were initially in a good mood but then felt yourself getting sick.

To protect both the shaman and the client during a cleansing session, it is important to open a window to allow the bad energy that is released from the client to easily flow out and escape into the universe, where it can be transformed. Or even better, the shaman can do the cleansing right in nature. Both of these measures protect the shaman from absorbing bad energy during the session. For additional protection the shaman can also blow or rub Agua de Florida on his or her hands or rub the hands in sea salt. This acts like a shield against negative energy, while allowing the shaman's energy to come through.

It is essential that healers practice regular energy-cleansing ceremonies on themselves and also in their home or office. A lot of healers, therapists, and others who work with many clients, after three or four years of practice, experience fatigue and are surprised to see their clients declining. This results from the healer not protecting and taking care of him- or herself.

Cleansing and protection are perfect methods for teachers and healers from all disciplines, such as reiki, massage therapy, dance therapy, and psychotherapy, But really anyone who works with other people, whether in an office or in customer service, can benefit from regular cleansing.

Here are the eleven stages of La Limpia as I understand them. Other yachaks may perform them differently sometimes as different people need different tools and techniques. (See full instructions on page 94.)

1. Greeting. Make the client feel comfortable and allow for time for energetic scanning.
2. Diagnostic and divination. Use a white candle and palm reading.
3. Consultation. Discuss the issues raised by the reading and learn the client's life and cultural point of view.
4. Energy removal and extraction. Use trago, green leaf branches, plants or herbs, blowing of fire, smoke, conch shell, and/or rubbing of eggs.
5. Rejuvenation. Bring in new positive energy to replace old negative energy, using Agua de Florida, red and white carnations or roses, and flowery aromatic oils.
6. Protection. Seal the physical body with volcanic healing stones, chonta spears, and tobacco.
7. Harmonizing vibrations. Use a bell and other musical instruments.
8. Calling back the spirit. Use a ceramic ocarina.
9. Embrace. Give a healing hug.
10. Candle blowing. Release the stored energy to the universe.
11. Final consultation. Discuss the client's experiences and visions. Give a prescription of rituals, ceremonies, and diets to be done at home.

SPIRIT POSSESSION

Often people contact me when they feel they are haunted or possessed by uninvited entities. These entities enter their bodies and crawl up and down, causing unbearable pains and instructing them how to think, act, and speak. These ordinary people feel hijacked by unknown forces and they are desperate. Most don't have any previous religious or spiritual backgrounds. Often they wonder how and why this could happen to them. They feel they were normal beforehand and want to know if they have lost their minds. They wonder if their experiences are real.

Are they imagining it? Are they acting out old traumas or re-experiencing them? Did they allow spirit to invade them or bring it upon themselves? And if so, are they responsible to discharge the entity on their own? All valid questions, I have learned never to contest their stories or experiences. They are valid, they are suffering, and they need help . . . fast.

In all human traditions stories are passed on containing accounts of individuals whose bodies and spirits were overtaken by evil spirits. There are Jinni stories of demons, or bad supernatural spirits, of the Arab and Muslim world. You can find many references to good and bad entities in the Christian Bible and in Tibetan, Buddhist, and Chinese mythologies. Jewish tradition claims two universal opposing forces: God and Satan. They are beautifully expressed in the Hebrew language: God's name is SHa DDaI and the word for "evil being" is SHEDD, which omits the letter *I—yud,* which symbolizes God—arguing that the state of evil is the lack of God's energy. Similar to reversing the English word live to spell evil. In Quechua, Kawsay means life-energy and Supay means non-life energy, or devil.

Spirit possession mostly happens to people who live in deep fear as evil feeds off fear and dark heavy energies. Their energy field shield—that orb of protection that surrounds each of us (just like the atmosphere protects the Earth)—is weakened and fractured by heavy negative energies. This can take the form of physical or emotional traumas, violence, intentional and unintentional curses, jealousy, and more.

Possession also can happen by being in harmful physical areas, such as homes where violence occurred or battlefields. Negative energies could be spirits of disgruntled deceased people, which attach to live people's energy fields or enter deeper and possess their bodies. Negative energy can also be manifested as a cloudlike dark energy that roams independently in the universe looking for frightened, vulnerable people to let them in through the cracks of their energy fields so that they can do evil's work. Evil feeds on fear and darkness.

SITRA ACHRA

My great-grandfather Mordechi Zundel Margolis, a *tzaddik* (righteous) kabbalistic rabbi from Kolono, Poland, devoted his life to the war with the Sitra Achra, an Aramaic phrase meaning "other side." He claimed that in the war between the dark and light forces, the dark ones wanted to divert him from the righteous path.

According to my great-grandfather, when God created the world, he gave people the freedom to choose good or bad. Choosing good means following God's ways, whereas choosing bad means distancing oneself from God and going after all kinds of earthly passions. Inside us we have our soul, which is our truest and purest manifestation. The soul wants us to live in tune with it, to be with God and do good deeds.

Beyond freedom of will, God created bad forces that exist outside human beings. According to my great-grandfather, these bad forces try to force a person to behave in ways opposite to his true soul— that is, to do bad things. These forces are what constitute Sitra Achra, the opposite of good. They seek to darken the world and consistently try to make a person choose bad over good. Because everyone has the power to choose good over bad, the bad forces are created so people can realize their inner powers. When we do not succumb to the bad forces or our negative impulses, we create happiness in the upper worlds and the light of happiness spreads down into the lower worlds.

Before I had a personal dramatic encounter with these forces,

I tended to look at them from a psychological or even so-called new age approach. I thought evil was illusionary and existed only because humans believe in its existence. I followed an approach that said spirits are neither good nor bad, benevolent nor malevolent, but can be so because of the projections of the mind. According to this approach, evil is a state of mind, and the key to deal with it is the power to change the mind by achieving a higher consciousness through various breathing or meditation techniques. Or evil can be diffused by using positive imagery and words and avoiding words that have negative connotations. Another view suggests that evil and suffering exist to help us learn life lessons and work through karma. From this perspective, bad and evil spirits are our most valuable teachers.

AN ENCOUNTER WITH EVIL FORCES

I have been going to the Amazon for fifteen years to learn from South American shamans. A few years ago, on the bank of one of the Rio Negro tributaries in the Brazilian Amazon, I took part in a sacred ayahuasca ceremony led by an Ipixuna tribal elder.

As the effect of the bitter brew took hold on me, I heard syrupy-sweet angelic sounds and then saw gentle-looking, whitish spirits hovering above me in a soft whirling dance. *This time it will be an easy ceremony,* was the happy thought that relaxed me. But that was not to be. After a while, those sweet spirits came closer and asked me to convert to their religious teachings. Naively, I politely refused, asserting my atheistic upbringing at the kibbutz where I was raised. But they kept sweet-talking me, promising salvation and all of my heart's desires in return. A red flag came up in my mind: who are these spirits.

Suspicion flowed into my body. They kept trying to tempt me. "If you follow our teachings, you will get what you want and become who you want to be." I became agitated. We started to verbally wrestle with each other.

"It's a trap, it's a trap, it's a trap!" I heard the ayahuasca spirit warn me. "Don't fall into the hands of evil. Look and see their real faces."

I looked up again and now recognized their true faces: they were contorted and ash dark with hollow eyes. I was taken aback. We began to argue again. They laughed acidly, saying, in a superior fashion, "You can't resist us. We rule millions of people around the world who follow us blindly!" We continued to wrestle for what seemed like a long time. At last, totally exhausted, I found my inner power and declared as loudly as I could, "I choose to follow the light! I'd rather give up my life than join you!" Again, I heard them ridiculing me. An inner voice came, doubting this statement immediately. I don't know how this idea came about but I found myself using all the energy I could muster in my shaky body to gather in the powers of light. Then I threw that energy toward them like I was a native warrior throwing a chonta spear on a group of ferocious wild pigs. I did not let go. I thrust it over and over again, until they slowly receded and finally disappeared into the dark void. My body relaxed. I was grateful to feel the reed mat under me.

I took a few deep breaths and looked up at the deep, starless sky. To my awe, just in front of me floating in midair was an unrecognized male figure. He looked like a spiritual teacher because he was engulfed in bright light. He opened his arms and said sadly, "The universal evil forces took over our ancient Hebrew spiritual teachings. They truly intend to conquer the world by fear and deceit." "Yeshua?" I asked.

At that instant I saw an extraordinary beam of light and love streaming from my heart toward this humble and loving fellow man. I felt great kinship with this man who was born and lived close to where I did. Then, I realized that a soft bright light surrounded me completely too. "You are part of me," he said kindly, and he slowly vanished.

My head began clearing. The bitter brew's effect slowly dissipated from my mouth and body. I heard the wind blowing through the jungle's leaves. Loud cicadas sang and the rhythmic cacophony of sounds of big toads and tiny green frogs filled the cooling night air. Bewildered by this unexpected vision and message, I lay on my mat for a long while mulling its meaning in my head.

THE SHAMANIC APPROACH

When I speak about evil spirits, I make a distinction between four types, which are slightly different in manifestation, origin, and experience. Though many times they can blend into each other, I still believe that it is helpful in shamanic work to make distinctions among them.

First, independent evil spirits come from a different realm than the one we live in and may take many forms, often of ghastly animal-like creatures. In the Tukano Amazonian language, they are called *akuras* or what we may think of as gargoyles.

Another type is simply bad spirits that are shape-shifting energy forms: they can be shapeless or can appear in human form. Sometimes these bad spirits are those of deceased people who were angry or frightened during their lives and died with those energies and have continued to spread them. Often people who are unhappy because of their "untimely" death continue to spread a kind of angry energy.

Third, there is bad energy that does not have a human appearance but is sent by humans to hurt each other, such as curses and the evil eye or sending out emotions like jealousy.

Last, these negative energies can also be found in certain geographical locations like land, springs, mountains, cemeteries, battlegrounds, and human habitats where traumas and violent activities occurred like wars, battles, murders, torture, and so on.

Accepting the view that evil can be an independent force in the universe may seem primitive and uneducated or a superstition from the past. Some shamanic traditions hold that there are no good or bad energies—just energy—and that assigning it is only a construct of our mind. But looking only for the light and not acknowledging the shadows and darkness is like denying the existence of night. One Amazonian tradition holds that several evil forces possess every person all the time. These can manifest as addiction, anger, sexual misdeeds, jealousy, lying, greed, stealing, and so forth. These characteristics are caused by an intrusion of negative forces, which can be removed by the local shamans.

SOME MODERN
EXAMPLES OF POSSESSION

In my workshops on shamanic self-defense, participants tell personal stories about their own encounters with evil spirits in various forms. In my healing practice I have encountered many clients who have suffered from some kind of possession. What follows are some examples of possession, with the names changed to provide anonymity.

Kathy, a professional in the world of finance, was hearing male voices who gave her misguided driving instructions, reprimanded her on her bad behavior, and sometimes punished her by preventing her from obtaining the jobs she was applying for.

Helen, a young beautician, claimed she was possessed by an evil entity that caused people she was in close contact with to have bad accidents.

Mary, a filmmaker, had her right hand shaking uncontrollably. The best neurologists in New York City saw her, and they could not find anything wrong. She believed it was caused by an evil intrusion. She was right. After a series of treatments, the hand stabilized.

Paul, an author, claimed evil spirits that resided in his stomach told him to hurt himself and mutilate other people.

Jane claimed she woke up at two in the morning to see a dark force in her bedroom, which then proceeded to strangle her. This vision repeated itself for a few months.

Brandon, a CEO for a high-tech start-up, encountered alien evil spirits during and after consuming ayahuasca. After repossession he resumed normal life.

Bruce, a practicing shaman, was having panic attacks due to the intrusions of negative spirits he absorbed during healing sessions with his clients.

John was cursed by his father, who told him from an early age that he was stupid and that he would never produce or do anything good or worthwhile. After a healing session, he went on to become successful.

Lidia was convinced a snake named Charlie had taken residence in her left leg and from time to time climbed up her spine. After his removal, she came back and asked to reinstate her friend. She missed his company.

People who experience possession report feeling engulfed by dark energy or a cloud that blocks them from moving on with their lives and prevents them from getting new jobs or pursuing their careers or finding the relationships they want. What makes seemingly sophisticated, educated, ordinary people living in today's highly sophisticated technological society and who are not necessarily interested in spiritual work experience these kinds of phenomena and seek the help of shamanic healers? Many of them come to a shaman after having given up on finding answers or help from Western medicine and psychiatrists. Some have been disappointed by the answers given by their religious teachers. When these sources do not reveal the source of their problems, they turn to shamanic healing as the last resort.

From a shamanic perspective, as I understand it, symptoms of spirit possession and bad energy can be detected in individuals and can also be found on a large scale in political parties and corporations and even in the spirit of an entire nation. When an individual is possessed by an evil or bad spirit, he or she will exhibit various physical, emotional, and spiritual patterns. The afflicted person may be unable to take charge of his life, feel shackled by unseen forces, and experience uncontrollable body shaking or a dribbling mouth. She may speak in tongues and have opaque eyes and sweaty sticky palms. He may experience paranoia, hysteria, a distortion of reality, soul loss, and a lack of empathy and may faint for no apparent reason and exhibit sudden radical changes in behavior. She may have a lack of reverence for universal oneness and unity and disrespect the well-being of Earth. I don't mean to imply that these symptoms automatically indicate possession, but I do find that one or more of these symptoms do appear in my clients who are possessed.

HOW TO DETECT EVIL SPIRITS

I asked Ipupiara about the nature of evil. He looked me straight in the eyes with his wise brown eyes and said, "It is hard to detect negative energy when it is not showing its real face, which it often does not do because of its deceiving and shape-shifting nature. Many times it appears as a force for good, love, and light. But evil or negative energy promotes suffering in others, which sometimes they accept in return for a temporary gain of money and power."

He continued, "It thrives on igniting fear, unleashing anger, creating separation and division, and calling for revenge. It creates helplessness and depression, mentally and economically. This heavy energy wants to slow things down and bring life to a stop. If not cleared, it seeps through our clothing and skin, into our mind, tissues, organs, and bones, resulting in sickness or even death.

"On the other hand, positive energy or light energy is easier to recognize because the forces of good tend not to harm anyone. This energy treats all beings with love and equality and shows reverence for Mother Earth. It is our role as shamans to remove negative energies and replace them with positive energies that restore health and balance to our clients' lives."

"But Ipupiara," I said, "why do some people do evil to others?" Ipupiara explained that "some people do bad things not because they were born bad—no one is—but because of the negative energy of outside forces they can't control, which they allow in out of fear."

THE POWERS
THAT SHAPE OUR LIVES

The ongoing battle between good and evil in the unseen worlds constantly shapes our experience of reality. We are all affected by it. These forces can be sent by other people, or they can come from greedy corporations, repressive governments, and radical political parties. These energies live in violent programs on television, the radio, the Internet, and other media. And as Ipupiara so wisely noted, evil can be difficult to recognize because it is secretive and elusive. Evil can impersonate the images of good and light, using deceptive words, such as *freedom, democracy, liberty, love, health,* and so forth.

So how can we decipher a message and decide whether it is good or evil? There is no way to tell immediately, 100 percent of the time, if a person, spirit, or message is good or bad. We need to pay close attention, read between the lines, and discover the real intentions of a person or corporation. We can investigate and determine whether an institution or individual is saying or doing things that are supportive of life or destructive to life, causing harm to others.

Good spirits never take over or possess a person's physical body, energy body, or mind. They do not cause harm. They support and guard us and treat all beings and nature herself with reverence. Good spirits work in light, transparency, and love.

Over the course of thousands of years, shamans from traditions all around the world have devised impressive toolkits for working with evil spirits. These include performing ceremonies and using herbs, minerals, stones, plants, eggs, candles, amulets, and so forth, as well as spiritual practices, such as prayers and energy shielding to protect people and their environments from the malicious, negative energies of evil spirits. We need to learn, practice, and become experts in these techniques and, by using them, cease to fear encounters with evil spirits and bad energies.

THE BAG OF BONES SHAMAN

All these healing tools and elaborate techniques are useful, but may not be as crucial as you might think in shamanic healing. Ipupiara once told me an intriguing story, which I have retold many times in my workshops to illustrate this point.

For many years he and his curandera (healer) wife heard of a legendary old woman shaman who lived a few canoe days away from their Taruma compound in Rio Negro. This old woman's reputation had spread all across the rain forest, and they were burning with a deep desire and determination to discover once and for all the secret of her mythical power before she passed away. So on one of their visits to their compound, they decided that this might be the perfect opportunity to visit her. After three grueling days of travel by canoe, hiking in the muddy flooded Amazon forest, and sleeping in different communities, they arrived at her community. They found her simple stilt wooden hut, and to their surprise, the old woman was already waiting at the top of the stairs as if she knew they were coming.

The old woman, wearing a simple T-shirt and a skirt, invited them to climb up the weathered cracked steps to her humble home. Following customary pleasantries, they settled in and began looking around curiously, expecting to see her altar with the sacred healing power items. But there was no altar to be found. Where is she hiding it? They wondered, glancing at each other. The only things in the bare room were a rough wooden sleeping platform and a bundle of old clothes tucked in the far corner. They looked at each other in amazement.

It was getting late; the sun had started to set over the trees in the west, and Ipupiara, who did not want to leave empty-handed, could no longer contain his curiosity. He took a big breath and at the right moment asked the old woman, "Please, can you show us the tools you use for your healing miracles, which you are so well known for?"

The petite, old "bag of bones," as Ipupiara described her, smiled a big toothless grin; her face, wrinkled like a dried raisin, brightened. She looked at him mischievously, a special spark in her dark eyes. Then she grabbed him by the hand and led him to an open window. There, pulling up her tiny body, she stretched across the windowsill and reached toward the nearest tree. In one quick movement she broke off a small twig, turned to Ipupiara, and said in her cracked old voice, handing him the twig, "Here, this is all you need." And she belly laughed so hard. Ipupiara and his wife were naturally disappointed. How did she outsmart us? They wondered.

In my usual skepticism, I naturally thought this was just a nice little story, a simple way to demonstrate his teaching. But to my total surprise, a few years later, while visiting Novo Airão, a small town located on the Rio Negro, where we went swimming with a group of pink river dolphins, Ipupiara met, entirely by chance, an old friend. He was an elder Waimiri-Atroari shaman who agreed to perform healing ceremonies for our small group on the deck of our boat. It was a courageous act of forgiveness by him, Ipupiara explained. In the aftermath of the collapse of the hydraulic dam the government built in the 1960s on their territory, this tribe swore never to engage with white people again. The dam collapsed on its first night of operation, taking with its gushing waters most of the tribe's population. It was their holocaust. You can't find this disaster mentioned in any official Brazilian records. More recently, the government had massacred some two thousand of them as they protested the building of BR-174, a new highway, and a new Balbina dam in their territory.

There he stood, a small man with bright narrow eyes, a big smile on his dark face, wrinkled by the unforgiving sun, wearing a large blue cotton hat. Holding a small branch in his right hand, he murmured a healing prayer and proceeded to carefully measure his client's body parts, calculating the proportions, the width and heights of his shoulders, the relation to the position of the neck, spine, and so on. He gave each of us an accurate physical, emotional, and spiritual diagnostic and proceeded to give us healing advice and instructions. We were all truly amazed by the simplicity and his accuracy. Above all I learned to trust Ipupiara's far-fetched stories.

LOVE IS ALL YOU NEED

Don José went a step further. He once told to me, "You know, I really only heal with one thing, with *love*." I looked at him in shock. I had been trying hard to learn all his complicated teachings for a few years by then. "Only love," he said and looked me straight in the eyes. "As the shaman stands in front of his client, he must remember that his client is also a manifestation of the apus [mountain gods] and the Great Creator. He needs to become the instrument through which flows the universal energy. The shaman must simultaneously be open and vulnerable enough to be intuitive and yet be as powerful as a warrior." He added firmly, "He must stop himself from making any judgment regarding the patient's character, body shape, or anything else and allow the energy of healing love to flow through him and direct him."

Ipupiara on another occasion said, "You heal with your heart intention, no matter what you know and how big a toolbox you've got."

THE RIVER AS TEACHER

A river is a perfect teacher to contemplate and learn about your life's journey. Some years ago on a beautiful afternoon at Harriman Park, in upstate New York, I sat on a black rock by a stream that flowed into the Hudson River. The clear, cold water rushed down the densely forested mountain. With happy bubbling sounds the water twisted and snaked its way between huge ancient black boulders and smaller rocks that had been brought down from far away by the melting glaciers of the previous ice age. Small pools and foamy waterfalls, dense green moss and white froth covered the bottoms of the small and large rocks as the water continued to flow, caressing the round pebbles and making sweet murmuring sounds. I observed the stream for a while. I closed my eyes and fell into deep meditation; the stream was teaching me.

Some fallen leaves and small branches floated downstream, and some got stuck and rotted in their place. Did they rot to give life for others? Was this their life purpose? Water never stops flowing by the formidable rocks; it finds ways around them and moves on or seeps into the earth. Those powerful hard rocks were polished, smoothed, and shaped by the never-ending stream of soft vulnerable water. Water collected in a muddy pool. I may not have been able to drink it, but it gave life to mosquitoes, frogs, dragonflies, deer, bears, and other forms of life. Would the trees be here if it wasn't for this stream? What was happening under the perfectly calm surface? Where did the water come from and where did it go from there, to the river, to the ocean, evaporating into thin air? What did it carry with it? Why did the stream never stop running? For me, the observer, the water was always flowing, but the single drop I just saw there was already miles away or even evaporated altogether. How did she feel?

Years later, near Manaus, in Brazil's Amazon at the Meeting of Waters—that sacred point to the local Manaós tribe where two colossal rivers, the Rio Negro and the Rio Solimões, the Amazon's tributaries, meet—I would learn other lessons on integration and unity with my Ipupiara and our small group. I was standing on a little river boat getting closer to performing the blessings ceremony for Yara, the Amazonian goddess of all water. Far out and all around us I could see broken trees, plants, and other debris from thousands of miles away being carried along by the two rivers' fast currents, as they sped on their way to unite with each other, creating a long wedding trail. The two rivers—the black one with its warmer, slower moving water and the red river with its colder water—journey side by side for many miles, slowly trying to merge with each other. They will finally succeed only when the two temperatures become one, the speed becomes one, and the rivers' colors become one. A great lesson and metaphor on how to unite our Western and Southern cultures together or any two cultures as a matter of fact. On the surface each of them looks awfully peaceful and lazy, but their undercurrents run swiftly and dangerously. Don't be fooled: deep under the calm surface in the muddy water dangerous fish with huge mouths and sharp teeth swim looking for prey. A fisherman was swallowed alive a week before our visit. Yara is known to be a temperamental goddess with mood swings that can change in a split second, creating a big storm with high, crushing waves. I experienced it a few times myself as she violently rocked our riverboat.

SAYING YES TO LIFE:
ABUNDANCE STARTS WITH YOU

Every shamanic tradition has time-tested techniques for removing the energy blocks that prevent you from connecting with the flow of life. Our fears, which come from negative experiences or beliefs, convince us that we are not capable, that we're inadequate or undeserving. We deny ourselves, often without even realizing it. Rather than allowing the universe to flow through us so we can receive the many opportunities it makes available, we stay stuck within our familiar limitations, like prisoners in our own comfortable cell.

Yes, abundance starts with you. By letting your river flow again, you will start to be in the flow of life and attract abundance to flow with you.

Here are some points to think about and work with. Be grateful and give thanks for everything that happens to you, both the "good" and the "bad." Both your "friends" and your "enemies" are your teachers; thank them for the opportunity they give you to learn more about yourself. Don't carry grudges; forgive yourself and others, especially your parents and siblings. Find what your life purpose is and what makes you joyful and passionate and pursue it with passion. Find faith in nature, in God, in the Great Creator. To flow in abundance is to share and give to others, to your community, and to those who need more then you do.

THE INCA WAY:
FAITH

Don José, after using the traditional diagnostic candle reading, often reprimanded those he diagnosed for their lack of faith. For indigenous people, living life without complete faith is unthinkable. Some clients asked, "Faith in what?" And he used to say, "Trust in the the apus, in Pachamama, and in Jatun Pachakamak."

"But how do you gain faith?" they asked in puzzlement. He then would look them in the eyes and with unflinching conviction in his fierce black eyes say, "You need to pray from your heart in earnest and concentrate on developing full trust in the universe." Come to think of it, no healing can occur without faith.

But what does it take to develop trust in a world where fear, deceit, and competition for power and scarcity of resources is the norm? Can you learn trust in the universe when we are so removed from nature ourselves? Can you learn to trust people who disappointed and harmed you? How can we learn that those obstacles are essentially opportunities for healing ourselves?

The Inca way of bringing healing and abundance into one's life is through an alignment with Earth, the universe, and our soul purpose or the mythic vision of our life. Only then can you enter into a balancing reciprocal relationship of give and take, in which you live in equilibrium and gratitude and trust Pachamama to truly provide you with all your needs.

In the Andes a special *despacho* ceremony is usually performed to bring about abundance by offering gratitude to Pachamama and the apus. In this ceremony participants place various grains, other food items, minerals, flowers, amulets, and personal prayers of gratitude or requests written on paper onto an offering blanket. At the end of the ceremony, the shaman wraps all the offerings in the blanket, making a bundle, and "dispatches" it to the spirits by burning the bundle in a fire or burying it in the earth. Fire ceremonies are used by many shamanic traditions to cast off negativity and other obstacles to make room for transformation and abundance.

Most ancient cultures had gods or goddesses of prosperity and abundance, for which they performed special ceremonies and prayers. Some are still celebrated, such as Saramama the corn mother; the Bolivian Ekeko, the mustached Andean god; the goddess Lakshmi, honored by the Hindus; the Celtic Letha; Isis in old Egypt; Frigga of the Norse; the Mongolian goddess Itugen—and many more.

The core shamanic belief is that the Great Creator created the universe perfectly and in full harmony. The universe can provide humans and all living beings with everything we need for our physical, spiritual, and emotional existence. Truly, there is plenty all around us to support and share with all beings on this Earth. So why is it that so many people live in scarcity? Why do some people lack trust in the possibility that we can all live in abundance and have to resort to hoarding fortune and resources at the expense of other humans and animals?

To believe in the unseen forces of life, you need to give up on existential control. You will gain emotional and spiritual freedom. It all comes down to faith. Scarcity comes from fear of not having enough for me to share with others and fear of poverty and of death. It leads to power grabbing, greed, and the distortion of reality. Scarcity is in the service and support of what we call the shadows or evil, the dark forces of the universe.

3
Healing Teachings, Ceremonies, and Techniques

The deeper we attempt to understand these processes using scientific tools, the more enchanting and miraculous this process reveals itself to be, and the appreciation of this ungraspable phenomenon only deepens our amazement and humility.

PROFESSOR RAFI MALACH

LA LIMPIA:
THE ENERGY CLEANSING CEREMONY

La Limpia ceremony can be performed indoors at the client's home or in the shaman's healing room or outdoors in nature at a spring, lake, or open field as circumstances dictate. Those participating in La Limpia undress, either fully or to their comfort level and stand in the middle of the room. It can also be done lying or sitting down if one is unable to stand for the duration of the ceremony. However the more the body is exposed the more the shaman is free to use all the elements in his toolbox, the more the skin is free to feel and absorb the healing, and the more effective it is.

The ceremony has eleven distinct sections, although it is not set in stone by any means. There is plenty of room for flexibility and add-ons of other procedures, depending on a client's needs and condition. Frequently, a shaman does not follow a described "schedule" but rather trusts her intuition and experience to lead her to do the right thing at the right time to get the best results for her client. Below are many possible procedures and pieces that can be included in La Limpia.

The Altar

The altar is the anchor, the source from which the yachak derives his personal power. Before starting the healing session he sets the right environment and ambience. He will wear his traditional white clothing, his colorful feathered headdress; he will hang the ceremonial necklaces around his neck and prepare and cultivate his *mesa,* or altar.

How the altar is arranged is very important and deliberate. The shaman spreads a red cloth the size of a bandanna on the table, as a symbol of Pachamama and strength. He then places a candle, his sacred objects (huacas), and healing stones in a predefined order on the cloth and sprinkles red and white carnation petals over the altar to bring it into harmony and balance.

First, the shaman blows trago and Agua de Florida on the altar's stones and other sacred items for clearing and appeasement and to feed them. She then opens with a chant and prays with palms open toward the heavens on her lap, summoning up the apus, the Great Spirit, the spirits of Imbabura, Cotacachi, and Mojandita Mountains, the sacred springs Magdalena and San Pukyu, the ancestors, and other spirits to guide her and help make the healing a success. She blows tobacco smoke on the healing stones to send for the spirits and puts her energy into them while she chants a tune. She calls the spirits while circling her right hand above the healing stones, first going clockwise, in the direction of the rising sun, to bring in the good energy. She then reverses direction, removing bad energy with her left hand. To keep the energy in the stones, she then pats the air above them. The right hand of the healer is used for healing and brings good luck, while the left hand is used for sending the bad spirits away.

The Chants: The Shaman's Soul Song

Chants are the shaman's soul song. The key that opens the gates to other worlds and his heart. Through breathing, the shaman vibrates the vocal chords, which frees his energy to move higher and connect with his helping spirits. The chant transports him into altered states of consciousness and delivers his power of intention for healing the client. Traditionally, the shaman sings, chants, or whistles continuously without a break throughout the duration of the healing ceremony. The chanting usually consists of a short, simple phrase or two and a melody that can easily be repeated. Customarily the words are requests from different spirits of the land, ancestors, or others to be present and help with the shaman's work or a request for protection and an expression of gratitude. The chant can also be sung in tongues—an unrecognized language—and it also can be whistled.

Chanting helps the shaman to concentrate on the task at hand; he shuts down background noises, removes his ego, and circumvents the gatekeeper of the logical mind. It helps the shaman be totally immersed and present in his sacred work. Most importantly a chant can be grounding, soothing, and reassuring for the client throughout the ceremony, helping her on her journey.

A chant can be passed down as a family tradition, received in a dream, transmuted in a vision quest, or given to the shaman by his power animal or spirit guides during a shamanic journey, or it can come in a moment of inspiration.

The Huaca: Sacred Object of Power

In the Andes, shamans believe that a shaman is as powerful as her huacas (*wak'a* in Quechua) and the intimate relationships she develops with them. These are the special natural or human-made objects containing sacred spirit that the shaman uses on her altar or those objects that she finds and enters into a special relationship with. In the Andes, typically, many shamans drew power from the volcanic mountains that surrounded them. There is no limit to what can be considered a huaca. It can be a physical object like a mountain, burial ground, spring, waterfall, rock, tree, cross, picture, stone, or sculpture of spiritual significance—or anything else that is a symbol of power and connection to spirit.

I once journeyed to retrieve a special huaca for a fellow traveler on a trip in Equador, a retired, white-haired, bubbly woman from California whom I had not met before this trip. We were sitting high on top of a burial mound, which is in itself a large huaca, near Hostería Guachala. It was early in the morning, and we were facing Cayambe, the snow-capped mountain in the east. As I closed my eyes to the sound of a drumbeat, to my utter surprise a small white poodle with dark bright eyes and a big smile jumped up and down on my body, licking my face with his sweet tongue, obviously happy to be recognized again. I was confused as this vision did not seem to merit, in my judgment, the seriousness of a worthwhile huaca. When I shared this vision with my new friend, she was overjoyed. It was her long-beloved dog who had passed away a few years ago. She told me about how she missed his love and wisdom as her teacher.

In another instance, when I journeyed to retrieve a huaca for another woman whom I had met at our New York Shamanic Circle's meeting, a plain white washing machine appeared. At first I rejected it as an object not truly worthy of power, but it kept on appearing. "Why? Because I am a woman?" she asked, visibly upset. Working through it, we later realized that the washing machine was a symbol and maybe an inspiration for the purification process she was going through in her own life at that time.

Consultation

Many well hidden and essential issues come to the surface during the divination readings, and they must be addressed immediately to give the client a framework, feedback, and insight into her life's condition. Here the shaman may act as a counselor, therapist, a life or business coach, or even a priest. Sometimes all the client needs on a particular day is to open her heart to someone who can truly listen to her.

Consultation time also gives a chance for the shaman and the client to get more familiar with each other, to share the client's history, and to create a deeper bond of trust between them. It is an opportunity to learn about the client's ethnic and cultural belief system. Many times a central issue can come up, which the shaman can address during the healing ceremony and then give the client an assignment for work at home.

It is crucial that the shaman withhold any judgment or preconceived ideas about the client's lifestyle and appearance and embrace him as a perfect manifestation of God's creation, as we are all mirrors of each other. Sometimes it can be helpful for the shaman to ask herself why the universe sent this client to her today, what lesson does the shaman need to heal through the client's unfolding issues.

Blowing Trago

La Limpia ceremony begins with blowing trago. The shaman puts a small amount of trago in his mouth under the tongue and blows out a soft mist with strong force on all sides of the client. Don't be discouraged if you are not successful the first few times. It takes years to perfect. As the stream of trago hits the bare skin, the client often experiences a sharp jolt of energy and gulps for air, which helps bring her consciousness into the present, releases tension, and connects her to nature's elements.

Made of pure distilled sugarcane alcohol, trago represents the sacredness of the unity of life. Through its roots the cane draws in water, the blood of Mother Earth, and other nutritious substances from Pachamama below. Through its leaves it absorbs Taita Inti's warm energy from above. This creates a perfect sweet union of the feminine and masculine forces in one cane that gives food and energy to our bodies. The plant then transforms the energies of the four elements (air, water, earth, and fire) into a pure sweet liquid of life that helps us transcend our everyday state of mind.

Additionally, trago represents the hard work it takes to plant, cultivate, harvest, and produce the sugarcane fields and bring sweetness to our life.

Connecting to this strong energy, the shaman can then perform the healing. It's good to drink a little trago before the healing begins to build up a strong energy. Some shamans believe that the more they drink, the less their ego is in the way of the healing process, enabling them to connect freely and directly with spirits, making them more powerful healers. Not all shamans agree with that assertion, as some don't believe in taking any consciousness-altering substances. Many of these shamans use herbal teas or spring water instead.

If you want a more logical explanation for this process, I found this explanation: the tiny alcohol molecule content of trago helps ionize the electromagnetic field surrounding the person by wrapping itself around the positive ions, thus neutralizing them. This makes for a more balanced energy field, which allows the client to feel refreshed and lighter.

Energy Removal

Using a shaman fan of dry palm leaves (*wayra* or *shacapa*), feathers, green tree/bush leaves, or healing herbs and plants, the shaman strongly pounds and brushes off the client's physical and energy bodies. She will start with the crown of the head and then go to the left hand, right hand, chest, abdomen, and all the way down to the toes to remove any effects or residue of bad energy. The rhythmic pounding and shaking also helps invigorate and awaken the body, creating a deep trance for the client that connects him through all his senses to nature.

Fire

Fire, the element of transformation, is used for severe mental or physical conditions and for getting rid of bad spirits, like attachment or possession. To do that, the shaman can choose a few ways. One way is to blow flames on the client's front and back body (also called focay). The shaman stands a few feet away, holding a burning candle in one hand, and then forcefully blows a stream of high-proof trago (such as Bacardi 151) through the flame in the client's direction. This is done powerfully with full concentration and healing intention. Sometimes the client holds a chonta spear on her shoulders to give extra space around her. Of course the client needs to be undressed so as to not catch on fire. Caution and judgment are needed here, as fire could be too strong a medium and could harm unaffected areas of the body if used improperly.

To apply fire to the specific areas that need cleansing, the shaman can blow high-proof trago on a eucalyptus branch, or any other green leaves, hold the branch over the client's candle until it catches fire, and then pat the affected area or wave the burning branch over the areas of the client's body that need healing. You can also use copal, palo santo, or any other sacred wood and surround the body with its flames.

Activating the Body's Energy Centers

I learned how to activate or deactivate the body's energy centers from Sarangerel, a Siberian shaman who passed on in 2006. I incorporate this practice in my La Limpia ceremonies as it helps open up the third eye, the heart, and blocked energies. To do this, the shaman holds a burning sage or copal stick and turns it clockwise nine times in the direction of the sun for activation of the crown, neck, heart, belly button, or sexual centers of the client while about a foot away from the body. To deactivate, the shaman repeats the same process, but turns the sage or stick in the other direction, counterclockwise.

Eggs

Eggs are excellent tools for healing aches and pains and for doing extractions. They are widely used throughout many cultures around the world. The egg absorbs energy through the seven thousand pores of its mostly calcium shell. These pores allow the developing embryo to keep the right temperature needed while exhaling carbon dioxide and inhaling oxygen.

All life begins with an egg. Bird eggs are the largest single living cells in nature and are a metaphor for the universal life structure. The yolk is surrounded by the albumen, the egg white, which is held by the protective membrane and shell; every cell in our body has a nucleus, plasma, and a protective membrane. The Earth too is made up of its interior inner core, its outer core's protective crust, and the surrounding shield of the atmosphere.

To dispel, collect, and extract bad energy that resides in the client's body, shamans use fertile organic brown or white chicken eggs. Brown eggs are sturdier and thus better suited to withstand the collected bad energies. It's quite rare to find in our urban culture fertile eggs, which carry new life force within them, so any organic free-range egg can do. It's also important to use both more pointed "male" eggs and rounder "female" eggs, to bring balance between masculine and feminine energies in the patient's body.

Holding an egg in each hand the shaman either softly rolls or vigorously shakes the eggs all over the client's body, concentrating on special areas that need attention, as seen in the candle reading and acupressure points. The shaman starts at the temples then goes over the forehead and moves all around the crown of the head and over the hair—clearing negative thought patterns. Next, he continues down to the torso, clearing emotions, digestive problems, fears, anger, and sexual energy. Next the eggs are shaken over the hands and legs, clearing circulation and improving the client's standing in the world. In clients who possess deep emotional or physical problems, the insides of the eggs often become hard as stones or crack open from absorbing all the bad energy. Sometimes an egg cracks or even explodes when encountering cancer, extreme tension and anxiety, or a bad injury. I have had eggs fly into the air as a result of energy being released.

The shaman can also suck on the egg forcefully in certain places to extract concentrated negative energy. The pointed side of the egg is directed toward the blocked area, while the shaman sucks strongly from the back. He then spits the bad energy into a garbage bag or bucket of water. This process can be repeated several times. It is important that the client remove anything metal from her person, such as rings or coins, before this process is done.

After the session, the eggs are put in a closed bag and buried in the earth in a special ceremony. Put the eggs in a hole dug in the ground and ask Pachamama to take the unwanted negative energy and recycle it. Cover the eggs with earth and step on them to break the eggshells, releasing the energy. For those living in a city, the eggs should be discarded as far as possible from the house to prevent the bad energy from returning and attaching to the shaman or the client.

Flowers: Carnations and Roses

The color and fragrance of every flower have unique vibrations and frequencies, which can interact with the body's vibrations for healing. Shamans use flowers to fill in the previously extracted bad energy and fill in the space with positive energy, a sense of harmony, balance, and well-being. Flowers can be used in two ways—by blowing or tapping.

The shaman collects a bunch of carnation petals from the altar and chews them, then fills his mouth with Agua de Florida and forcefully blows the mixture over the client's entire bare body. The shaman then asks the client to rub the mixture forcefully into her body, starting with the legs and going up to the stomach, heart, face, hair, and back. This mixture must stay on the body until the next day.

An alternative is to rapidly tap a bouquet of mixed red and white carnations on the body, starting with the head and moving down to the feet. Often you can bring positive Earth energy up the client's body by pulling the flowers upward from the feet to the heart. Doing this cements the power and fragrance of the healing flowers. Sometimes the shaman asks the client to ingest the petals at the end of the ceremony.

The colors of carnations have importance and symbolism too. White carnations represent the male energy (ideas, spirituality, upper world), red represent feminine energy (passion, blood, lower world), pink evoke feminine youthfulness (combination of both), and yellow represent Taita Inti, Father Sun, sunrise as a new beginnings. White, red, pink, and yellow roses can be using in similar ways.

Healing Stones

Smooth black volcanic stones are the source of the shaman's power and his personal pride. They are used to absorb negative energy from the body, for grounding, and for creating a strong protective shield around the client before sending him home. These stones hold the power of the four elements. They are formed from magma that has erupted from

Earth's core and risen to the surface, undergoing changes in temperature and pressure, which cause it to cool and solidify. For this reason, they are believed to have the highest condensed energy and density. Volcanic stones are often passed on in the family or given as gifts between shamans. Traditionally a shaman can't purchase these stones; they must be passed down to her or given to her.

The stones are either naturally polished by the elements or by a craftsmen to give them a smooth surface, as they are used on the client's skin and as a mirror reflecting the flame during the candle diagnostic reading. Each stone must have its own name and assigned gender, which is revealed to the shaman in dreamtime by holding it in his left hand throughout the night. The stone's name must be kept secret and not be revealed—not even to the shaman's spouse, children, or any other shamans.

With a male stone in the right hand and a female stone in the left, the shaman first clicks the stones together in a circular motion around the client's head to shake and remove whatever negative energy is left. Simultaneously, with one hand on the front side of the head and one on the back side of the head, the shaman lightly rubs the stones, one from the forehead to the crown of the head and the other from the base of the neck to the crown of the head. Then the shaman moves the stones around the entire head and temples to seal the head from negative energies. He then presses hard with one stone under the shoulder blades and one opposite that on the chest and moves the stones up to the base of the neck to release hidden muscle tension there, which holds fear. Then he lifts the client's arms and using one stone on each side presses them firmly in circular motions two to three inches under the armpits to stimulate the horary cycle point to activate the release of hormones that promote well-being. The shaman also makes a circular movement on the lower back in the triangle above the buttocks to release tension and fears. He finishes by moving the stones in rings around the neck, chest, stomach, pelvis, and each hand and leg to create a solid field of protective energy and a strong shield. When this is all done, the shaman blows trago on the stones on all sides to clear them from any negative energy.

The stones must be taken care of periodically by immersing and washing them in sea-salt water to remove static negative energy. They also need to be recharged: they are set outside at noon to absorb the masculine energy of the sun and are put under the light of a full moon to absorb feminine energy. They also need to be fed every Tuesday and Friday at sunrise with trago, chocolate, candies, and fruits. From time to time they need to be given a rest and removed from use.

The Chonta Spear

I believe that the Quechua yachaks of the Andes adopted the chonta spear as a healing tool from the Amazonian basin tribes, such as the Shuar. You can easily spot the chonta, or Brazilwood, tree, as it rises above the jungle's canopy. It is sacred to the Shuar as a symbol of life and abundance. It's incredibly useful and essential to their diet and unique way of life. Its red sweet dates (*chontaduro*) and their inner palm hearts (*palmitos*) supply the Shuar with plenty of delicious and important nutritional food and cooking oil. The fruit's harvest time beginning in March marks the Shuar's New Year and is a time of a weeklong special celebration with community dances and the drinking of *chica* (a fermented drink made of the chonta fruits). Because of its height, width, and straightness, combined with it sturdiness and moisture resiliency, the tree is used to build dugout canoes and for making weapons like the long hunting and ceremonial spears, blowguns, bows, darts, and daggers. That is why in the healing ceremony the chonta spear comes to represent the character of the fearless, unbreakable warrior.

Toward the end of La Limpia healing ceremony, the client closes his eyes and is given a chonta spear to hold vertically, away from his body in his two hands. The shaman asks him to merge with it and feel its raw power. Then the shaman pushes strongly on the spear a few times so that the client can find his balance, ground himself, and find his inner core power. Then the shaman can switch the spear horizontally across the client's chest and push again a few times. Then the same is done vertically behind the client's back so he can find the strength of his spine. Last, the client carries the spear on his shoulders.

During this process the shaman blows tobacco smoke on the client's palms in each stage to bring spirit's blessings to the client's inner warrior.

The chonta spear or a dagger is also used to sever invisible attachment cords that connect between the client and her other relationships (parents, siblings, coworkers, etc.) The shaman does this by moving the spear in very quick cutting motions all around the client's physical and energy body and above the head. It also can be used to send blessings to the heart or other parts of the body by the shaman pointing the spear to the chosen area and blowing tobacco smoke over the spear in the direction of the client.

I love the e-mail I received from one of my regular clients describing her experience with the chonta spear.

"Journey to your power animal to find your inner warrior. Find out how it will manifest itself." I had no idea what this meant, but I closed my eyes and stood in front of you with complete faith. . . . When you finally took the stones from my hands I thought, as if I were some kind of expert, "Oh it's over now. Time for the Agua de Florida." But instead I heard you fumbling around to my left for something else. I kept my eyes closed. . . . I trusted you, but I had no idea what could possibly be going on.

You put the chonta spear in my hands and began to push . . . barking at me not to let you move me. This is when my journey began. I was there in the room listening to your orders; doing the best I could against your strength considering I was having shoulder surgery in two weeks. But I was also in the jungle flying with my Hawk. I always had been capable of flying with him, but now he left me on the ground at the base of a tall tree that was branchless until the canopy spread out high above me. At the base of the tree I saw that the dirt had animal prints that circled the tree around and around. Up above, Hawk was calling me to climb the tree to be with him. I protested saying that I can't possibly climb this tree, but he kept calling me over and over . . . mocking me that I was scared and weak.

But then I felt as if I was changing. I started pacing around the base of the tree looking down at the earth at the paw prints. Then amazingly, I saw that my feet were the paws. . . . I was making the tracks. I had become Black Panther. So I looked up at Hawk, reached up my powerful paws with enormous claws that dug into the tree and I began to climb. I could see my shiny black fur and bulging muscles that pulled me higher and higher.

All the while I was conscious of your voice continuing to bark, "Stand up straight! Use your spine!" and I worked hard to push against you. I felt tears fighting out of my eyes in anger, and refusal to fail, determined to show you my strength. You put a drum above my head and began to drum loudly. There was more smoke . . . more chanting . . . more pushing from all directions . . . and in my journey I continued to climb.

When you finally took the spear from my hands, I was shaking and buzzing, and covered in sweat. "What just happened here?" I thought as I panted to catch my breath. I was grateful to finally receive the sweet smelling Agua de Florida in my hands, so I could rub it on my skin and cool down. I walked on shaky legs to sit down, and all at once my shoulder began to scream in pain. I looked at you and said, "How did I do that? My shoulder didn't even hurt."

"Because that wasn't you . . . it was your inner warrior," you said, with that familiar smirk on your face and a look of satisfaction.

Smells and Aromatic Oils

Our nose is a perfect and powerful vehicle to deliver messages to our brain through our chemosensory receptors of smell. It connects us to old, sometimes forgotten memories and buried feelings and brings them forward to the conscious mind. It can instantly transform the mood of the client and improve overall well-being. Shamans use fragrances throughout the ceremony—the smoke of different woods or herbs, rum, flowers, cologne, and aromatic oils. I use crushed fresh mint leaves, which I grow in my office, to help people release nausea, relax, and promote deep breathing.

Don Jacho Castilo, an Ecuadorian yachak, performed a special healing ceremony using aromatic oils. He poured a few drops of aromatic oil on the client's palms and directed him to rub it in a very quick and strong manner, while concentrating on the thing he wanted to manifest in his life, such as love, health, courage, work, abundance, friendships, and so on. He asked the client to say what he wanted loudly with deep conviction as he bore witness to it. The patient then brought the palms of his hands to his nose, inhaled deeply, opened his arms in a wide circle above his head, and exhaled. He repeated this pattern twice more, embedding his wishes in his subconsciousness. (The same process can be performed to do a shamanic journey as the client inhales the oil's scent to receive messages from spirit.) Don Jacho then rubbed a drop of aromatic oil lightly on the client's third eye in a circular fashion nine times at the end of the ceremony—"to seal the ceremony," he said.

Tobacco Smoke

Tobacco has a bad rap in our culture due to industrial and commercial abuse, which has caused addiction and diseases. But in many societies, such as those in the Amazon and Andes and among Native Americans in North America, wild tobacco is considered sacred. Tobacco is recognized as an important healing plant used in community and healing ceremonies as offerings to spirit. It has purifying properties; when drunk as a tea it purifies the digestive system by eliminating bacteria and viruses and by changing an acid environment into an alkali (antacid) or base environment. As a smoke, it creates a protective energy field around us.

Tobacco smoke is used toward the end of a ceremony. By blowing pure tobacco smoke on top of a client's head, the shaman is letting the smoke rise to the heavens as an offering to spirits and as an omen to foretell a good healing outcome. She then pats the crown of the client's head to hold that energy down. The shaman may sometimes blow smoke through a special stone with a small opening in its center to the third eye, heart, or other areas she feels might need this.

Next, the shaman lays a chonta spear across the chest or points it toward the heart and blows tobacco smoke on it. She repeats this process on the client's back and sometimes on other parts of the body as needed. Often times the shaman will blow tobacco smoke on her hands and body at the end of the ceremony to cleanse herself and get spirit's blessings.

Sound

As mentioned earlier, throughout the ceremony the shaman uses the sounds of his chant, songs, prayers, or whistles to transport himself and his client into a state of shamanic consciousness or dreamtime. After the protection has been completed, the shaman will rapidly ring a small, high-pitched brass bell starting at the top of the head and then all around the person's body. This is done to harmonize, align, and balance the vibrations of the physical and energetic bodies.

At the very end of the ceremony the shaman stands behind the client, and with a small, high-pitched ceramic Ukus (ocarina) he blows a high, sharp sound, like a birdcall, behind the client's head. This opens the top of the head, the crown, to the heavens and brings back the client's traveling soul. This is sometimes called spontaneous soul retrieval.

Water

Cleansing in natural bodies of water, such as springs, rivers, lakes, oceans, and waterfalls, is an essential part of any healing. Water is considered the blood of Mother Earth, the basic element of all life as there is no life without it. It purifies the body and soul. Water connotes emotional flexibility and flow, like a river. It is the feminine energy that connects us to our deep intuition and Grandmother Moon. Water comprises 60 percent of our body weight and, as Emoto has proven, its structure can be altered by the energies projected upon it.

Before performing a healing ceremony near a water source, it is important to first identify the gender, either male or female, of the body of water. Two sources of water, one male and one female, must be selected. The ceremony needs to be performed at both sources so balance can be achieved and maintained.

First the shaman invites the client to stand with her in the water.

The shaman opens the ceremony with a chant and a prayer and asks the water spirit for permission, coaxing it for cooperation in the upcoming healing. She makes offerings by blowing trago on the water, sprinkling carnation flowers on the water, and blowing tobacco smoke.

Some spirits that reside in water can be benevolent, but others can be malicious and even deadly, so it is important to either appease them or leave them alone. Don José told me of one particular male spring on Imbabura Mountain that took the lives of many people because they did not make offerings and respect it.

At the end of the ceremony the client cups water in the palms of his hands and pours the water six times over each of his shoulders, beginning with the left side, and then pours water six times over his head and six times down the front of his body.

Following La Limpia Session

Following La Limpia session it is important but not mandatory that you observe these points to maximize the results of the healing:

- Take some time to rest before driving home; walk or spend time in a park to ground yourself. The session could make you feel tired and sometimes disoriented.
- Do not schedule any big social activities; do not interact with other people's energies.
- Do not shake hands on the day of your session to prevent the transfer of negative energy by others. The palm is supersensitive as it contains thousands of nerve endings.
- Do not take a shower or bath until the following day.
- Avoid sexual relations or ejaculation for at least three days following the session.

For the next two weeks avoid these foods:

- Avoid caffeine in all its forms, like coffee, chocolate, and green or black teas, as it overly stimulates the nervous system.

- Do not drink alcohol as it raises the sugar level and suppresses awareness.
- Reduce consumption of sugar and yeast.
- Do not eat pork, beef, and poultry meat; fish and seafood are best as they are easier to digest.
- Avoid spicy food as it raises the stomach temperature and acidity.
- Drink chamomile tea at breakfast and before bed.

All the foods eliminated above create heat, excess acidity, and nervousness in the stomach and nervous system. So eat balancing alkaline foods. Drinking chamomile tea after you wake up and before bedtime has many health benefits including help in sleeping, relaxation of the digestive muscles, and an overall calming effect.

For one of my clients, not drinking his morning coffee was a sticking point. After one of our sessions he stopped smoking three packs a day as I was able to extract his grandfather's addictive spirit out of him. Yet, one day I met him on the street. "You know, I really want to book another session with you," he said. "Well, I'm always available. Send me an email," I told him. "I can't," he said shaking his head. I was puzzled. "I'm afraid you will make me stop drinking coffee too," he seriously answered. He never came back. This is how seriously people get addicted to coffee.

DIAGNOSTIC AND DIVINATION READING

Shamans and healers the world over, from all traditions, are able to observe their prospective client's physical, emotional, and energy bodies and then decide what is the best way to bring about healing. By entering nonordinary reality, shamans are also able to receive hidden knowledge and messages from the spirit world in order to help them reveal the root causes and nature of their client's health, relationships, beliefs, and spiritual conditions.

These tools and techniques are essential for a successful healing and can be taken with you and used on your own with family, friends or private practice. Read on and practice these techniques so you can develop a deeper connection with your spirit helpers, learn to scan and perceive the three bodies, develop intuitive hands, read candle flames and stones, and more.

Here are a few techniques for diagnostics and divination from different traditions. All can be very surprisingly accurate and useful, and one can choose to employ one or more at the same session.

To be able to give a good reading, make sure you remove your ego from the process. Become a hollow bone, a transmitter of knowledge, a messenger of spirit with no stake in the results. Trust spirit or your intuition that the messages you receive, either by hearing, seeing, feeling, or simply knowing, are the right ones for your clients.

Seeing or Gazing

"Seeing" through the physical body—like an MRI—is a useful technique any time during a session or just in life in general and particularly before a session begins. In many instances, using seeing, I am able to see the reason why people come for the session. Sometimes spiritual entities appear with them, like unborn children, current family relatives, and distant ancestors. Sometimes I can see their physical illness (or that of a relative) before they have a chance to explain.

To see, stand before your client, so you can see him entirely. With a soft gaze observe the person's entire energy field and then travel inside the body to the inner organs, legs, knees, and feet. Try not to focus on the client's physical features and details of clothing. Start from the space above the head and proceed all the way down. As you precede you can try to "see" with closed eyes too. Take mental notes of the messages you receive from spirit. If a certain area needs more attention, ask your spirit guide what's the source of that condition. Share the insights and answers with your client later.

Energy Sensing

Prepare by washing and strongly rubbing your palms with Agua de Florida or water or shake them well to activate them. With open palms, move your hands lightly over your client's body. The client can either be standing up or lying down. Start slowly, from the crown of the head to the toes. Allow yourself to sense fluctuations and changes in temperature throughout the body, which can indicate energy blockage due to physical illness or emotional trauma. Close your eyes and let your healing intuition and your spirit guide give you their messages. You might feel some of your body parts hold tension or pain; it might be a message from your client as well. Sit in front of your client and discuss what messages you receive in their entirety, without your interpretation and censorship. You will be surprised.

Palm Reading

This is an ancient art form of interpreting the lines, skin condition and texture, and coloring of the palm; the shape, length, and size of the fingers; and the shape and condition of the fingernails. This technique needs extensive learning, although some people can intuitively read hands. Many cultures have different points of reference in palm reading, and probably they are all correct, as long as they can help people find happiness and direction in their lives. My readings are usually not intended to read the future, but to help a person find her life purpose and direction and understand her key characteristics so she can make the right choices that support her life purpose.

There are four types of palms correlating to the four cardinal elements: earth—those who are practical, often physical workers, bakers, gardeners; air—poets, philosophers, and thinkers; water—those who are emotional and artistic, often teachers and politicians; and fire—those who are passionate, leaders, and impatient. On each side of the base of the palm you can find the sun mount (masculine) and the moon mount (feminine) and a valley between them, just like the Maya built their temples, and there are four other mounts under each of the fingers.

Each finger represents different attributes related to a different planet: pinky represents Mercury—communication and sexuality; ring finger, Venus—the emotions; middle finger, Saturn—intellect and logic; and pointer finger, Jupiter—authority and leadership. The thumb shows how well you handle your life in general. There is more to it of course as we look at the major lines (head, heart, fate, and life) as well as sublines, which show information about relationships, health, intuition, healing, success, and so forth.

Egg Reading

A fresh brown or white egg is rubbed softly all over the client's body to accumulate his physical and emotional energies through the egg's porous shell. Start from the head and go downward. Once done, crack the egg into a clear glass of water. Let the contents of the egg settle for a few minutes and don't move the cup. Look at the textures, forms, white filaments, bubbles, colors, and consistency and location of its yoke and other parts floating in the water.

See if there is any blood or dark spots, indicating possible illness. Cloudy water indicates signs of mental confusion. Bubbles on the white filament and above might be negative energy directed to your client and you will need to perform a strong cleansing. Spots on the yoke mean that someone is directing evil toward your client. Most importantly use your intuition to interpret the meanings while sharing and discussing them with your client. Once the reading is done, dispose of the contents in the bathroom and flush twice (or see earlier discussion of egg reading in La Limpia for alternative disposal, page 101).

Bones, Stones, and Rock Reading

To diagnose if someone is possessed, ask your client to hold a small bone between the two index fingers of his hands. If the bone is stable, there is no possession. If the bone starts to rattle and shake uncontrollably, it is a sign that the person is possessed, and you have to proceed immediately with depossession. If the bone shakes on the left side, it indicates a problem or attachment of the feminine energies. If the bone shakes on the right side, it indicates a problem or attachment with masculine energies.

Bones and/or stones can be tossed by the shaman into the air to fall randomly on the ground. The shaman interprets the bones or stones by the way they scatter on the ground.

In a rock reading, the client chooses a rock, about the size of an orange, and holds it in his palms for a few minutes and concentrates. Then the rock is laid in front of the client, and the client then describes through association to the shaman four of the rock's characteristics on its topside—its scratches, colors, textures, and cavities; for example, "I see a moon and a road that splits in two opposite directions. There is a large tall mountain, and I also see a shape of a lion." These marks represent the client's future. The shaman writes the information down.

Then the client turns the rock over and describes what he sees on the bottom side and again shares four images with the shaman. The underside represents the client's past. The shaman writes down what the client says and then uses those images to interpret the symbolism and metaphors relevant to the client's life.

The Shamanic Journey

A shaman journeys into nonordinary reality to obtain answers to specific questions on behalf of her client or for herself. During the journey, she receives revelatory knowledge from her power animals or other helping spirits. Shamanic journeying can be done with the help of a fast; with monotonous, rhythmic drumming, rattling, dancing, or chanting; with the help of plant medicine; or by simply concentrating and connecting directly with spirit helpers. All are equally effective tools.

Often, a client's spirit helpers—deceased ancestors, living family members' spirits, and other entities that are surrounding the patient's body energy—come to assist the shaman in her work. They are the message carriers for the client and sometimes can offer profound insights and various instructions on how to heal the client's condition. Some entities will be revealed as faces floating in a gray cloud. Some are as clear as a hologram and appear fully embodied, and some are only a brush stroke of black or white cloud energies.

Spirit can be a great help and provide accurate information if you surrender to it without fear or judgment. Share with your clients all the details, without censoring them, as the information you'll be receiving is not meant for you and can be better understood by your client. Essentially a shaman is like a pizza delivery boy who doesn't judge his customer for the toppings he chooses.

Shamanic language and communication is not linear; it is the language of poetry. Pay attention to the flow of symbols, colors, sounds, smells, and textures. Write down your journey and try interpreting the meaning or lessons behind the visions. Each person will perceive visions and messages differently. Some see visions, some feel things, some hear voices, and some know. You may not see something because of an unconscious fear of knowing. Remember, the world is as you dream it. It is okay to make it up or go with your imagination, as everything comes from our mind's eye anyway.

Some people have several strong detailed journeys and then have a dry spell, with no visions. Don't panic; it's okay. Continue to try without reprimanding yourself. The visions will come back again. A friend from my shamanic circle had his first vision of his power animal after six months of trying, and he eventually became a great journeyer. We all experience times like that; we are not machines after all.

How to Journey

In a quiet place, lie down, close your eyes (it helps to cover them), let your body weight merge with Earth, and take a big breath. As the drumming begins (if you don't have someone drumming for you, you can listen to a CD of drumming or simply lay your hand on your heart and concentrate on your heartbeats), imagine a portal from which you can enter into the lower world. It's best if you can chose a place you know intimately. It could be a cave, a tunnel, a crack in a rock, a well, or an elevator. Enter it and start your journey into the depths.

Walk toward the light at the end of the tunnel and emerge into a different landscape: it could be a jungle, desert, or mountaintop. Look around. You'll see a variety of animals that can fly, swim, walk, or crawl.

They are all equally qualified to be your guide. When you see an animal that you feel a strong affiliation with, tell him who you are and the purpose of your journey. Ask the animal if he is willing to be your teacher. If he agrees, ask him what is it that you need to learn from him at this particular point of your life. If he says no, ask him to lead you to another animal until you find one. Like watching a movie, allow him to lead you, but do interact and ask questions. Don't be shy: spirit prefers that.

When the drumming rhythm changes, it is time for a callback. Wrap up the conversation, wherever you are (you can always come back to it later), and thank your power animal. Then a very rapid drumming will begin, and you start your journey back. Retrace your footsteps (try to revisit every detail of your journey) and emerge through the tunnel into the portal you came from, back to our reality. Bring life back to your body, move your toes and fingers, and stretch out. If you do not understand your vision or might have other questions, journey again and ask your guide. Questions need to be open-ended, not yes-no questions. They need to be when, where, what, how questions, such as: What do I need to know? How should I resolve an issue? Where should I go?

Animal communication can also happen with words or through body language gestures or telepathically. Each animal has different medicine and embodies qualities that may be similar to yours or may be those you aspire to. Try to understand what the animal stands for. You can also search the Internet for different interpretations from different sources and traditions for your particular power animal. Feel which interpretations speak to you the most.

You can have more than one power animal. Sometimes a specific animal will show up to work with you on a specific issue. Animals come and go according to your own needs at particular times of your life. People always ask me if power animals are real or if they are a construct of our subconscious mind or imagination. Since I "see" them as holograms above people's heads while they journey, they are real all right. But truly it is not important. Surrender to the magic.

Upper world journeys are done to meet a teacher in a human form.

They are done in the same manner, except that you need to look for a portal to lead you to the skies above, like a tree, a vine, or even a chimney. Some say there are different layers and different teachers on each. Do a journey and find out for yourself. On my first journey to the upper world at a Michael Harner workshop I found a teacher. He had not yet crossed over. I was really upset to receive it; I wanted my money back. But he had great wisdom to share with me at the time. The teacher was O. J. Simpson. Go figure.

Journeys to the middle world attempt to connect you to the spirit and consciousness of objects in nature and the cosmos, such as trees, mountains, rock, rivers, home, stars, and even your iPhone. Everything has spirit and can be a teacher. You can use your power animal or teacher to do journey there, or let your intuition lead you.

Candle Reading

Candle reading is an ancient pre-Incan diagnostic technique widely used to this day by the yachaks of the Andes. The client rubs an unlit white candle (not in a candle holder) made from natural beeswax or paraffin over his body to let the candle absorb physical, emotional, and spiritual problems or issues he has come to heal. He stands with eyes closed and starts from the top of the head, goes over the face, and then proceeds to the left and right arms, and finally to the rest of the body, going over the legs and back, while strongly concentrating on the issues and problems he has come in to resolve. When this process is done, he cups the candle in his palms and strongly blows on it three times, transferring his healing intention and spirit or soul to it, and then hands the candle to the shaman. This process can also be done independently as it is a great way for negative energy removal. In this case light the candle and let it burn all the way down.

The shaman holds the candle lightly at the bottom, lights it with a match, and starts reading. The client can interact with the reading. The shaman must hold the candle lightly so as not to transfer his energy to it. The candle should not be lit by any other source to keep its purity. If the flame goes out, it may indicate that the client possesses heavy, bad energy and even suicidal tendencies. Do not use the same candle again; begin the process from the beginning.

After the reading or at the end of the healing session, the client blows out the flame with a prayer to release the issues and problems he came with into the void and then buries the candle in the earth to allow any bad energy to be transformed by Mother Earth. During this reading process, the shaman looks at the overall picture: the strength and size of the flame, the colors' proportions, the relative position of the wick, the shape of the wax drippings, and the flame's textures, shapes, and movements.

Colors in the Flame

Blue: Blue represents the power, strength, and vitality of the mosocnina, or sacred fire. This fire is formed by the infusion of oxygen with fire. The blue dimension, on both sides of the wick, reflects the strength and tenacity the person possesses (more is better). If one side is bigger, it represents an imbalance between the material world and the spiritual world. If the blue climbs up the wick to the top, the person is spiritually inclined or developed. When you see a blue tone above the tip of the wick, it represents active night dreams, visions, or spiritual engagements. A dark spot or cloud at the bottom of the blue region represents digestive problems, which may be related to fear caused by early childhood trauma. The point between the blue area and the wick is called *uru daurwa:* it is the gateway where spirit enters into the candle's flame according to a message I received in dreamtime from my late teacher Ipupiara.

Purple: Place a finger behind the blue region. If it turns into light pink or magenta, the person is holding resentment and feels victimized. She thinks, for example, that life is not fair and that she has been unfairly targeted by negative events. If the color is a strong reddish-purple, it may indicate feelings of strong anger or rage.

Yellow: This color represents the sun energy. It is a good energy, indicating clarity and an overall good disposition and balanced life.

Orange: The combination of yellow and red indicates strong, intense, active positive energy and well-being.

Black, Dark Gray, and Brown: This is a sign of negative energies—the darker, heavier energies. If you see these dark colors around the person's body (represented by the wick) or around the head (tip of the wick), it indicates persistent negative thoughts, such as self-deprecation, stress, and fear. If the darkness is at the bottom of the flame, in the blue area, it indicates indigestion and energy blockage by fear and trauma.

Often, you may see shapes or waves of grayish-colored energies within the yellow and orange flame areas. In my experience, those are images of either living people or of departed ancestors that reside within the person's energy orb. Concentrate on them. Try to "see" and communicate with them. They are there to bring messages to your client.

Green: Green hues represent envy and jealousy, as in "green with envy"; the jealousy could be felt or directed to the client by other people or within the client toward others. A lighter, brighter green can also be a sign of attracting money or abundance. Use your judgment.

Red: Red tints or spots in the flame's orb or the wick can indicate strong anger, which can lead to acute health problems, sometimes even cancer.

The Wick

Look at the wick as a representation of the client, who is surrounded by her own universe (the flame). The posture of the wick reflects the person's physical and emotional condition. Is she standing straight and tall, or is she short, squeezed, bended, or folded? Is she reaching outside his own world or staying alone and lonely in the center? Examine the wick's irregularities and bumps along the wick's length. You might be able to tell if the person has spine problems, upper or lower back aches, neck aches, thyroid or heart issues, constipation, or digestion problems.

The wick's top represents the person's head or mind. If it is ablaze, larger than normal, it represents an overactive and strained mind. If the wick's top is divided into a few strands of flames, the person is torn, debating options, and is confused. If you see flickers of light coming from certain locations along the wick (spine, heart, appendix, lungs, womb, etc.), they symbolize health problems in those areas, such as infection, ulcer, pain, and so on.

The Flame Shape

If the flame is burning evenly and steadily and is round in shape, the person is pretty balanced. If it is long and tall, it indicates that the person is reaching toward more spiritual life goals. If the tip of the flame is zigzagged, it indicates a belief in and connection to extraterrestrials. He may have experienced alien abduction, had dreams or just fascination. Jumping and leaping flames demonstrate struggles to overcome obstacles. A candle flame that rises and flares constantly indicates nervousness and unsteadiness. A halo around a well-proportioned flame demonstrates that helpful spiritual entities surround the person. If the base of flame is unusually high above the wax, it means that the person is aloof and may not be grounded.

The Wax

A deep curved pool under the flame indicates a deep mental depression. If it is flat, the person's feelings are normal. Wax that drips and overflows indicates sadness and crying. Wax that hisses, crackles, and pops represents emotional instability, nervous energy, and the possibility of spirit possession.

Eyes

Light a candle and bring it close to your client's eyes. Pass the candle flame from side to side of the face. Ask the client to follow the flame with her eyes. If the eyes are expressionless and lifeless, it is a sign of soul loss, possession, or attachment.

PROTECTION TECHNIQUES

Physical Processes for Protection

Smudging

Smudging with smoke composed of a variety of plants, herbs, resins, and minerals can be an exceptional energy purifier for your body, home, or office. Spiritually, smoke summons helping spirits; it represents the transformation from solid matter to spirit, as the smoke ascends and disperses into thin air. Physically, smoke captures negative energy particles in our illuminated body or habitat spaces and in hard-to-reach places, then removes and transports them to the heavens to be dispersed. A recent article in the *Journal of Ethnopharmacology* notes that smoke can disinfect the air from a variety of dangerous airborne bacteria, hence it has considerable healing properties.

The most popular plants for smudging are white sage, sweet grass, lavender, rosemary, valerian root, and other aromatic plants or trees, like cider, pine, palo santo, and copal. For body purifications, start from your head and go down to your toes. You can disperse the smoke with your hands or with a feather through an open window or into a candle flame. You can also scatter these plants and minerals around the house for protection against evil spirits.

House Energy Cleansing

Clearing bad air, negative energies, ghosts, and good and bad spirits from the house and workplace is as important as clearing one's energy field. Often it is important to clear the owner's energy right after you clear the space. This ceremony uses almost the same tools as in La Limpia. The premise of this common practice in South America is that humans, animals, or any object leave energy footprints wherever they go. Sometimes deceased people's spirits still stay at the place of their death, as they are not willing to move on. Negative energy is heavy, stagnant energy that stops the flow of life; it sinks down. If not cleared, it can bring bad luck, fear, sleeplessness, and sometimes violence to the people in the house or building.

I have seen a lot during the years I have practiced this form of clearing—from an old sailor who hanged himself in the attic of an Amsterdam warehouse to a group of electronics thieves in a store in Queens; from an abusive Middle Eastern husband to an uncooperative Indian wife; from a murdered young woman's ghost that crossed my room at 2 a.m. in Ecuador to a loving old couple who lived a full life in Queens, New York; from a killing dungeon in a Lower East Side restaurant's basement to an unsuccessful factory in Long Island; from a cheating famous Brazilian healer to a Middle Eastern woman who vowed to ruin my client's business. All past events that were later confirmed. And the effects of the clearings brought back harmony and good luck and changed people's life.

The shaman's role is to shake and invigorate these negative energies to move them out of the house and return the house to harmonious balance and flow. Throughout the ceremony the shaman chants or whistles an icaro (soul song, or prayer). If a house has multiple floors, the shaman starts from the bottom and moves up. Windows are open to let the negative energies and smoke out.

Here are the instructions:

1. As you enter the house, stop, gaze at the surroundings, breathe in, and then close your eyes. Ask your spirit guides to inform you on what is going on in the house. Wait a few minutes for a vision or answers. Sometimes spirits and events will be shown to you as holograms. Pay attention and go to the places your visions lead you when you do the clearings.

2. Start by setting up your altar, light a white candle, and call the four directions and your spirit guides (I usually call my teachers' spirits in this and the other world) for help with healing intention and prayers.

3. With a bottle of trago walk all around the rooms and blow (camay) through your mouth (preferred) or a spray bottle in the corners, under the bed, closets, kitchen, drawers, and behind the doors, in all the hard to reach places where stagnant energy lies. The trago's alcohol molecules neutralize the positive ions in the air to create a more balanced environment.

4. Light a sage stick (or any other plant), walk around the house, and

fan the smoke where there is stagnant energy. (You can use your hands or feathers.) The smoke removes old energy and kills airborne bacteria.

5. Walk around the house and vigorously click two healing stones with your hands to shake up old energies. You can also clap your hands or use a rattle.

6. With a bottle of Agua de Florida walk all around the rooms and blow through your mouth (preferred) or a spray bottle in the corners, under the beds, in closets, in the kitchen, in drawers, and behind the doors, in all the hard to reach places, to bring good energy.

7. Walk around the house and puff tobacco with the blessings of spirits.

8. Walk around the house and ring a high-pitched bell to harmonize the house vibrations.

9. Gather with your client around the altar. Hold hands and pray with intention.

10. If you were called because of relationship and love issues, put red, pink, and white rose petals on the bed after the cleansing. Ask the owner to have fresh roses by the bed and to take a rose petal (boil them for five minutes) bath before she goes to bed.

Sea Salt

Sea salt is a natural detoxifier and absorber of negative energies from your skin and your environment due to its hygroscopic ability. It is used in almost all healing traditions around the world. Rub your hands and your entire body thoroughly with salt, or take a handful of sea salt and add it into a bath. Place small bowls with sea salt and water (no need to change the sea salt, just replenish the water) in the corners of your house, under the bed, or in your office. You can also use sea salt without water. You can also fill up a bowl of water, add handful of sea salt, and dip your hands in it for a few minutes.

Corn Flour

This is excellent for the removal of strong emotional problems and spirit attachments. Rub it over the entire body. It has the ability to repel negative energies and is used to create a protection circle around a person, a house, or sacred spaces by forming a line that bad spirits will not cross.

Coal

Coal absorbs negative energies and is also perfect against bad dreams or nightmares. Grind the wood coal, preferably from a ceremonial fire, wrap it in natural fabric, and tap it over your body or put it under your pillow to help you sleep as it absorbs reoccurring bad thoughts and nightmares.

Baths

Take a handful of sea salt and pour it into your bathtub and lie in it for twenty minutes. You can also add a spoonful of baking soda. If you feel strong negative energies around you, take a bath with sulfur (put sulfur sticks or powder in water overnight then pour the water into the bath). For heavier attachments add six drops of ammonia to the water. Boil a bunch of rue leaves for five minutes and add them to your bath. Some shamans recommend taking beer baths.

If you do not have a bathtub, you can fill a bucket with water. Pour water using the palm of your hand, six times over your left shoulder, six times over your right shoulder, and six times over your head. Do it with prayers, pure intention, and concentration. Repeat it on three consecutive days, starting on Monday. You can also dip your hands or your feet in a bucket of water with sea salt. Do not soap or shower after the bath.

Sweating It Out

Spending time in a sweat lodge, steam room, or a sauna can remove toxicity and purify your body, emotions, and soul. Sweating lets the negative energies on the surface of the skin and in the deeper tissues pour out of the body.

Blowing of Sugarcane Rum

Put a small amount of sugarcane rum (trago) in your mouth, under your tongue, and blow it out forcefully on yourself, on others, or around the room in a strong intentional blow. It needs to be sent as a strong but soft mist. It will ionize and rebalance your energy body and surroundings.

Eggs

Containing thousands of pores in their shells, eggs are excellent for absorbing negative energy. Roll an egg over the entire body, starting with the head and moving down to the feet; concentrate on an area you feel needs more attention. You can also suck the bad energy out in your mouth and spit it into either water or a plastic bag. To dispose of the egg, it is recommended to bury it in the ground with a prayer.

Feathers

Use feathers, preferably condor, eagle, or wild turkey, to remove stagnant negative energies. Start at the crown of your head and move all the way down to your feet. Let the feather guide you to feel energy blockages just like dowsing; feathers represent the element of air and the clearing wind.

Stones

Brush healing stones, preferably black lava stones, over your body to absorb negative energy and create a protection shield. You can also hold a stone in each hand or put them in your pockets for grounding. For your home and office, clap the stones around the room (or rooms), especially in the corners where stagnant energy congregates. After using them dip them in sea-salt water or blow sugarcane rum on them to cleanse them.

Green and Black Candles

It is believed that wax absorbs negative energies. Rub a green candle over your body, preferably on your bare skin. Green repels akuras—evil spirits—who cannot tolerate the color of life and growth. Start from the crown of the head and go all the way down to your feet. Light the candle, place it on a safe surface, and let it burn all the way down. If you experience stronger spiritual attachment, rub a black candle in the same way; black is the color of evil energy cast on you. Light it and turn it upside down. Hold it, and let it burn down completely. For better results do this ceremony for both candles on three consecutive days or as long as you need it.

Amulets

Amulets can be a piece of jewelry or an object made from stones, seeds, metal, or coins. Amulets sometimes contain words or prayers. They are worn and are created to protect the wearer from harm and evil spirits. They are sometimes blessed and imbued with the power of a shaman. Wear a protective charm, pendant, or bracelet on the left hand, the path to your heart, or over your heart.

Mirror

Wear a mirror or any reflective metal surface over your heart center to deflect a negative energy attack back to the aggressor and to disperse it into the void.

Plants

Plants absorb negative energy and produce negative ions for air purification. Place various plants with large green leaves—such as aloe vera, banana, arrowhead, evergreen, dumb cane (*Dieffenbachia*), geranium, and dragon plant (*Dracaena*)—around the house and on windowsills. A very important plant in South America is rue, also called ruta or ruda (*Ruta graveolens*). It has a very distinct repelling smell and beautiful small yellow flowers that need lots of sun. Plant it in the entrance to your home and place it on your windowsills. It is believed to shield the house from jealousy and envy of neighbors and passersby. Tap a small branch of rue all over your client's body; if the plant dries or dies, it is a sign that your client possesses large amounts bad energy. Boil a branch and add it to your bath or spray or clean your house with it.

Nature

Spend some time in nature. It contains and emits negative ions, which counter the positive ions we are surrounded by in our homes and offices in our digital society. Walk barefoot as much as you can, hug a tree, or sit with your back to a tree trunk; it will absorb your negative energies. Some people find it helpful to be buried in soil or sand for a few hours or overnight; the soil clears your energy and grounds you. Stay by or swim in a lake, river, waterfall, or ocean. Encase your body with plants and green leaves, as they repel evil spirits. You should also wear green clothes for the same reason.

Handshakes

Do not shake hands with people who you believe are angry and depressed as they are carriers of negative energy. With more than a million nerve endings and receptors in the palm of the hand, shaking hands acts as an energy transmission between two people and could be contaminating. Sticky, sweaty palms can indicate an emotional nervousness, fear, and disturbance.

Sulfur

Sulfur—a foul and smelly crystal—removes emotional problems, hexes, and attachments and frees one from enemy attachment cords. You can roll sulfur sticks over your body, preferably on your bare skin, from head to toe. You can also soak sulfur for twenty-four hours in water and add it to your bath. If you do not have sulfur sticks, use sulfur powder encased in a fabric pouch and tap it on your body. Sulfur can also indicate signs of possession. Hold a sulfur stick in both hands. If it breaks, it is a sign of possession. Bring the stick to your ears and if you hear cracking and hissing sounds, it is a sign of emotional disturbance caused by entities.

Protection Stones

There are many stones and crystals that have protection energies. They can absorb or repel negative energies. Stones such as black obsidian, black tourmaline, black onyx, and apache tears can transmute good energy. Wear them around your neck, carry them with you, or place them around you in your home or office.

Other Physical Protection Tips

- Hang a wind chime on your window or in your garden; the sound will send away bad spirits.
- Spray holy water, a salt-and-water mixture blessed by a priest or spiritual teacher.
- Hang a horseshoe above the door.
- Hang a garlic garland above the main door and other doors; no one can stand against its strong smell and purifying powers. You can also wear it around your neck.
- Take a sunbath for ten to fifteen minutes each day; negative energy shies away from the light.

Psychic Processes for Protection

- Be aware and alert. Use your intuition to spot danger and bad energy from people around you who are angry, agitated, or depressed and will suck your energy out of you and also from negative places.
- Sit quietly. Take a few deep breaths. Close your eyes and visualize yourself surrounded in a bubble of light. Or imagine a source of white light above your head; encase yourself with this protective light.
- A heart filled with love is the strongest protection. Send love to your nemeses; it is hard to do but necessary to give them gratitude for their teachings and not hold anger and resentment in your heart.

ADDITIONAL HEALING TIPS AND CEREMONIES

Aloe vera: To protect your home, place pots of aloe vera around the house. It is also excellent for digestion, acid reflux, and skin problems. Just peel a leaf and use its gel.

Aromatic oils: Rub oil on the body or inhale it. These oils carry antioxidant, antimicrobial, and anti-inflammatory properties and can sometimes reconnect us to old memories. For example, eucalyptus oil is excellent for opening breathing channels. Rosemary is good for mouth care, anxiety, depression, asthma, and so on.

Bee stings: Lay a bee on an aching joint and allow it to sting. The sting will bring a rush of blood to the area as the red blood cells attack the bee's poison. This helps relieve pain in rheumatic and arthritic conditions. *Cautionary Note:* It's best to ask an expert to do this procedure and you must make sure you are not allergic to bee stings.

Cedar leaves or pine needles: Cedar and pine are good for bone strengthening or for use as an antiseptic. Take baths. Boil the leaves or needles for five to ten minutes, and pour the water into the bath or on yourself. Do not rinse; towel dry. Repeat this bath for three consecutive days.

Chamomile: This herb is excellent for relaxation. Drink it as tea or take a chamomile bath. Valerian can also be used for relaxation. Boil the herb for five minutes, and pour the tea into the bath or on yourself. Do not rinse; towel dry. Repeat this bath for three consecutive days.

Charcoal: Place a small pack of crushed natural charcoal (preferably taken from ceremonial firewood) under the pillow before returning to bed; the charcoal will absorb negative energy and thoughts. You can also place it around the house and office to absorb negative energies.

Grapes: On New Year's Day, take twelve round red grapes; hold each one and concentrate on what you wish to have in the new year. Eat each one slowly, enjoying the sweetness.

Natural Needles: Natural needles, such as a porcupine quill or cactus spine, are good for awakening the nervous system and stimulating the inner organs for health, especially during pregnancy. Gently tap the needle on the bottoms of the feet and the area around the ankles. (See further instruction on page 136.)

Red and Pink: If you are a single woman looking for love and relationship, wear only red or pink underwear. No black. In addition take baths with red, pink, and white rose petals (boil them for five minutes before placing in bath) for a month either before you go out in the morning or before bedtime.

Rocks: To calm an overemotional state, put small rocks in your pocket or hold them in your hands.

Roses or carnations: For marital problems, boil red and white rose or carnation petals for five to ten minutes. Stand in the shower or bath naked with your spouse, facing each other. Take turns pouring the flower tea over each other. First pour over the right shoulder, next over the left shoulder, then over the head, and finally over the entire body. Let your bodies air dry. Repeat on three consecutive nights. These flowers are also good for attracting love or support a new relationship. Boil red, pink, or white rose petals, or a combination of carnation and rose petals, for five minutes, and pour this flower tea into a bath or pour over yourself, from head to toe. Do not rinse. Take this flower bath for twenty minutes on three consecutive days (or when needed). It is recommended to also spread red petals on your bed and put fresh roses in the bedroom.

Sangre de drago **(dragon's blood):** Rub this antiseptic sap from an Amazonian tree in circular motions to heal mosquito bites, skin rashes, or cuts. Drop three drops into a cup of water and drink to clear digestive problems and your blood.

Stinging nettles: This plant has many health benefits. Beating it on the naked body and joints promotes blood circulation and relieves arthritis, inflammation, and acne. Use it as a tea to stop infections, internal bleeding, diarrhea, and other digestive problems.

Urine: Urine is good for cancer tumors, acne, and kidney problems. For cancer, collect the first urine of the morning of yourself or preferably of a young family member. Dip a cotton cloth into it and put it on the stomach for one hour. Do the same for acne, collecting the urine of yourself or a young family member and put the cotton cloth dipped in urine on the acne spots. For kidney problems, collect your first urine of the morning. Soak newspapers in the urine, wrap the papers in a towel or plastic sheet, and put them on your lower back. Doing this will warm the kidneys.

Yellow: On New Year's Eve and Day, wear yellow underwear and put yellow flowers around your house to ensure that you have a good year. Yellow represents Taita Inti, Father Sun, and is a symbol for a new energy and the beginning of new life.

Soul Healing or Retrieval

All across shamanic traditions soul loss—the wounding or fragmentation of a person's soul as a result of sudden fear, trauma, abuse, accidents, war, conflicts, and so on, especially when it's suffered at an early age—is seen as a leading cause of illnesses, immune-system deficiencies, and all-around dysfunction of physical, emotional, and mental well-being. Sometimes a soul loss can accrue in other ways, such as soul stealing by another person to keep part of that person's power or through soul exchange, for example between lovers or parents and children to become dependents. Sometimes a soul loss did not even occur in this lifetime but is hidden in a long-gone past life. I have witnessed this for some of my clients—as a fallen knight in England, a woman healer in France, and sex worker in India. If not treated, soul loss can result in a permanent condition, repeating dysfunctional patterns, and avoidance of engaging in life's opportunities.

What is a soul? No one can tell you for sure. But we all know it as that unattached, energetic essence that is free to move in and out of our bodies and makes us uniquely ourselves. You might want to think of soul healing as trying to find and fit lost pieces of yourself as you put together the jigsaw puzzle of your true self. If you could find those missing pieces, you would have a complete beautiful picture. I can't imagine there is anyhthing more healing and satisfying than that.

How can you tell if you have a soul loss? Many of my clients complain of feeling detached, empty, devoid of purpose; they feel they are living an aimless life and are unable to concentrate. Some experience deep depression and have suicidal thoughts. Many simply have suffered a memory loss of crucial years from early childhood. Some say that their heart is closed and they can't feel love. As one client said once, "I feel as if there is a hole in my heart."

Usually the symptoms are the result of unconscious impulses to deaden one's feelings to avoid the unbearable pain of a trauma and still be able to carry on with life's challenges. It is nature's sensible survival strategy of the psyche, but it takes a toll on our vitality and health as we move on with life.

There are many shamanic approaches to healing this condition. Most famous is to journey into the spirit world with the help of a spirit guide, witness the trauma, track the "lost" soul part, communicate with it, convince it to return to the client, and blow it back to the heart and crown of the head to reintegrate it back into the energy body of the client. Each culture or individual shaman finds its own unique way to perform this retrieval, and no one way is better than another. Some societies perform this special healing ceremony during certain times of the day, such as at noontime, while others do it at midnight, when they believe the cosmic portals are open. Sometimes it can be experienced spontaneously, with or without the direct help of a shaman. This happened to me in a sweat lodge ceremony on the Big Island of Hawaii, and it sometimes happens to my clients during cleansing ceremonies. Spontaneous retrieval could also happen on a mountaintop, in the midst of a remarkable landscape, or while listening to music, where the detached soul part feels safe to reconnect and return to be seen.

In the aftermath of a successful soul retrieval ceremony, people feel more grounded, full, happy, content, and courageous and are better able to engage in their lives. As one of my clients said, "I experienced a second joyful childhood, one that I was never able to know before. I finally experienced a carefree childhood and found the child who is loved."

Soul Integration

To fully benefit from this work, the client must go through a conscious process of uniting with that lost part and becoming its caretaker. Nobody can do this for her. Additional shamanic journeys may be needed to meet and welcome back the lost part. The client may need to conceive of specific ways to heal the old wounds. It also helps for the client to be aware and acknowledge the changes that happened in her life in the aftermath. The client needs a supportive group of people who can be with her as those changes happen, and she needs to consult with the shaman about how to make true physical changes in her everyday life that will reflect and honor her newfound part. I ask my clients to adopt a doll for two weeks, or more, that can remind them of themselves at the age that the soul loss occurred. I ask them to take care of it around the clock—talk with it, feed it, bathe it, and take it to work—as a constant reminder. It works miraculously.

An e-mail I received from a client beautifully described her experience with another form of soul retrieval.

I was amazed that you saw in the candle's flame a deep trauma around the time I was three years old. At first I could not remember it. Then it hit me. I was only two and a half years old when my parents came to the US from Israel. My mother was depressed and realized she needed help. She checked herself into a hospital and put my sister and me in an orphanage. You asked me how I felt when it was time for me to leave the orphanage. I told you that I always felt that I left a part of me there. I felt abandoned and alone. It was interesting because I have always felt like a part of me was missing but couldn't figure out how to become whole again

I agreed to try an exercise that you suggested. I closed my eyes and you led me to meet myself as that little girl in the orphanage. It was very sad as I remembered many of the details. By the end I adopted her and promised her to love and protect her. We did another exercise that brought me to when I was around five years old. I introduced the two and a half year old me to the five year old me and we hugged and kissed and cried. You asked me if I wanted to leave the orphanage with her, and I said yes. We held hands and together we walked out of the orphanage building and she brought me to a park where we played and we were very happy and carefree. From the park, the two of us travelled through the years until the present and I put them in my heart and we hugged and cried. We became one, a whole person. You suggested that I would open my eyes. I told you that I was never able to have a regular childhood.

Before I left your office you asked me to buy a small doll that looked like me as a child and carry it with me for two weeks and do all the things that I missed out on doing as a child. Take the doll everywhere, you said. At first it felt strange but in a good way. By the end of the two weeks I noticed a big change in me. I was happy and at peace. It was fun, my husband went along with it and he enjoyed having little me with us. He understood that this was something I needed to do.

Aztec Seeing and Body Work

This simple-to-use Aztec modality of bodywork can be used for diagnostic reading and for healing. It allows the shaman to tap into the body-stored memories and bring them to the surface and enables him to have a dialogue with his client. It allows you to unravel incidents, relationships, and memories the client never previously shared or told you about. At the same time it resets and rebalances the client's mind, body, and spirit energies. As we lay hands on the client's body we have to listen deeply to our hearts, trust our intuition, and have faith in the process. In this modality you and your client are encouraged to simultaneously share what each of you "sees" or feels as it is happening. Here is how it works:

The client lies on her back—this can be done fully clothed—either on a table or on the floor. Do an energy clearing first, using either your hands or feathers, to remove any negative energy the client might have. Lay your left hand, the receiving hand, lightly on the client's navel. Close your eyes and open yourself up to receiving messages from spirit, either by feeling or through visions or call on your power animals for help.

The navel represents the center of the universe and the cradle of life. More than seventy thousand nerve endings in our body converge in the navel, which makes it a very sensitive center. In addition, at the center of our palm there are more nerve endings than almost anywhere else on the body (except our feet). This meeting of these two highly sensitive energy centers in turn connects us to our nerve impulses, which come from the brain. The nervous system is what is responsible for our emotions and thoughts as well as our body movements.

Feel the energy that flows into the palm of your hand and listen to messages that come in. Keeping your left hand on the client's navel, lay your right hand lightly on her solar plexus, or heart center, and wait for messages about the overall emotional energy. Then move your right hand to the right side of the navel, the place that represents the body's masculine energy, and wait for messages about the masculine experiences of your client (father, brother, and other males); share what you are experiencing with your client. Now place your hand below the navel, at the center of the life force, or sexual energy, and share with your client. Then to the left side, which represents the feminine energy of the body, and share with your client. The purpose of this is to check in all four directions, going in a circle around the navel. It also simultaneously rebalances the client's energy body, even if you do not see anything.

Once you are done, proceed to lay both hands on the chest to feel your client's breathing and then lay your hand around the neck and share any information you gather from this with your client. Put your left hand under the head, and the right hand on the forehead. Listen and share. Put your left hand below the jaws and right hand over the crown. Listen and share. Then move behind the client's head and lay one hand on each of the temples. Listen and share. Then keep the right hand at the crown of the head and lay the left hand on the navel. Listen and share. Then move your hands to the feet, knees, and pelvic. Listen and share along the legs.

Finish by going back to the beginning: place your left hand on the navel while putting your right hand on the solar plexus and around the navel. Sense whether the client's energy has changed.

During this entire process the client and you should be sharing your visions, thoughts, memories, and feelings. As I said, I use this technique often and am able to see relationships between the client and her parents and best friends and connections with the client's home, place of work, and many more associations.

Takuma Needles

From the Brazilian Amazon, this technique can be used for diagnosis and for healing. The takuma is a palm tree that bears sweet date fruits. To protect them from sweet-toothed monkeys and other animals, the tree ingeniously grows long and very sharp black needles in dense rings around its trunk. For our purpose you can also use any other natural sharp needles, such as porcupine or hedgehog quills, cactus spines, and so on.

Our largest organ, the skin, wraps around our entire body and is equipped with millions of sensory receptor cells as an alert system or survival mechanism (fight or flight). It responds to external stimuli, such as touch, temperature, and pain, by creating electrical impulses throughout our body and sending them to our brain. Needles can stimulate, invigorate, and activate the body's entire nervous system by sending messages to the spinal cord and brain, and from there to the organs that need healing.

The client lies on his stomach, preferably fully naked or wearing minimal underwear.

Start with energy cleansing. Blow trago or brush the client with green leaves or feathers. Close your eyes and, starting at the head, pass your two hands lightly above the entire body; feel temperature differences, which may indicate places of energy blockages (cold) or infection (hot), and listen for your spirit guide for messages about your client's condition. You can share what you sensed with the client, if you like, but it's not necessary.

Stroking with Needles

To prepare ask the client to remove his clothes and lie on his stomach. Hold two needles, like chopsticks, in one hand. Then follow these instructions:

1. Start at the left shoulder and lightly stroke the needles down the shoulder blade's triangular area in a succession of four or five strokes, proceeding from the top of the shoulder down, making lines from the left side to the right side. Repeat three times.

2. Move to the right leg. Stroke the needles down the thigh under the buttocks to the knee, in a succession of four or five strokes, proceeding from the top, making four or five lines from the left side to the right side. Skip the knee area and continue down to the ankle, and then stroke the sole of the feet. Repeat three times.

3. Go to the right shoulder blade and repeat the same as you did on the left shoulder blade (step 1).

4. Now go down to the left leg and do the same as you did on the right leg (step 2).

5. Stroke below the back of the neck between the shoulder blades' triangular areas in a succession of four or five strokes, proceeding from the top of the neck down, making lines from the left side to the right side. Repeat three times.

6. Stroke the whole length of the spine until you reach the crease of the buttocks in the lower back. Repeat three times.

7. Stroke the triangle of the lower back in a succession of four or five strokes, proceeding from the top of the triangle down, making lines from the left side to the right side. Repeat three times.

Poking with Needles

Important note: do not puncture the skin. This technique is not like acupuncture. Tap the needles lightly; for some sensitive people it could be quite painful. Here is how you proceed:

1. With your two needles poke along the sides of the spine, going from the buttocks to the neck. Repeat four times.

2. Then with one needle poke lightly a few times at the lower back triangle.

3. Then poke the needle on the back opposite the heart.

4. Then poke the upper triangle below the neck and between the shoulder blades. (Those two triangular areas of the upper and lower back are very important, as the muscles there usually clench when a person feels threatened, fear, anxiety, or stress. As the muscle contracts and expands, you can help it release negative energy.)

5. Take a moment and poke the needle behind each of the earlobes to release brain endorphins. You are now done with the back and can go to the palms of the hands.

6. Start with the left palm. Use a sharp needle in a circular motion going clockwise, in the direction of the sun. Start with the sun mount under the thumb (masculine energy). Then do the moon mount under the pinky finger (female energy). Then proceed to the center of the palm and then to each side of the palm. Next do the areas below the fingers; tap each of the fingers. First go to the pinky (Mercury), which symbolizes communication, intuition, and sexuality. Next go to the ring finger (Venus), which represents emotions and creativity. The middle finger (Saturn) is logic and intellect. Then to the index finger (Jupiter), representing authority. The thumb represents the overall condition. Finally, do the point between the thumb and index finger and proceed to the side of the palm.

7. Do the right hand in the same manner. When you are done with both palms, go to the soles of the feet.

8. Start with the heel and go in a clockwise motion, going over the sole and toes and the sides of the feet.

9. When you are done with the soles, poke under each of the ankle bones, on both sides a few times. If the ankle is swollen, it indicates problems in blood circulation and kidney function. It is also important to activate this area as it connects to women's fertility organs and thus the ability to get pregnant.

10. To finish the process, blow Agua de Florida on the client, pat her body with flowers, use your stones to create a protective shield, and ring a bell to harmonize her energy.

Anytime you see your client's body react to the poking, it is a sign that the inner organs, the spine, or other body parts need special attention and healing. Find a foot and hand chart on the Internet to learn the locations connected to each of the body's organs. Be aware that not all charts are the same as different cultures and schools map the body differently; you will soon discover what works for yourself. Even if you don't know which of the organs you are working on, the result will still be beneficial for your client's health.

Some people react violently: the body may jerk or twist. Don't be afraid; let them release that pent-up energy. Some will feel pain but will not express it; encourage them to express it and release it. It is important to give them permission to react, or they will hold or block their emotions. I urge them to breath deeply, yell, scream, or, if need be, curse me. It helps in the energy release. Sometimes a layer of sticky sweat will pop up and cover the client's hands, feet, or the entire body, which is an excellent way for the body to release bad toxins. Ask them to drink a lot of water right after and on the next day.

Sometimes after a treatment, a client may feel tired and emotionally drained. Ask him to refrain from social activities and sleep or rest as much as he can, as the body needs to readjust. Like this e-mail from a client: "I could not sleep, except finally at 6 a.m., I fell asleep for 4 hrs. Even with the lack of sleep, I feel better today—somewhat more energized and calmer at the same time." Or this e-mail from another client: "I've had a much more intense emotional reaction to this last session than to the previous sessions. Lots of grief, despair, sadness, helplessness . . . so I'm just giving it as much room as possible. And by last night I had a migraine. Interesting!" I especially like this e-mail, which I received from a client who suffered multiple weekly migraines: "This really amazing thing happened: yesterday was the most stressful day I've had in years, and I feel absolutely exhausted, but I have no headache. This is a miracle." Another client wrote: "I felt so balanced today during the takuma needles . . . at peace with them . . . accepting of their pain, and grateful for the relief they bring me for the left shoulder."

Drum Healing

Much healing is achieved by the administration or guiding of energy vibrations into what we call the physical and energy bodies, which creates an harmonious flow. Drumming vibrations can penetrate deeper and with more precision than rattles, other musical instruments, or vocal sounds. Drumming vibrations penetrate the skin, go into our tissues and inner organs, and go even deeper into the skeleton and bones— our structure. The vibration of drums synchronizes the brain faculties, helps us enter into higher awareness and consciousness, releases emotional stress and traumas, and boosts the immune system.

Today there is a lot of scientific research into the effect of drumming on our brain and its healing benefits. Most shamanic traditions use a drum for communication or ceremonies but not always specifically for healing. The frame drum came to us from the East, from Siberia and Mongolia, and traveled to the Americas with human migrations. Drums carry a great deal of symbolism. The circular wooden frame covered by an animal skin represents the skin of Mother Earth, thus of the feminine energies. The circular shape represents the complete life cycle as there is no beginning and no end, just like the circle we sit in around a fire. We are sitting on the Earth at the same eye level as equals. There are no students, no teachers. We are all one. We are all the same. The drumstick represents the masculine energy that awakens the heartbeat.

We bring all of those elements to healing when we drum over the client's body. Drumming isn't about the power of the banging; it is about listening carefully to each of the Earth's heartbeats as we communicate with her. Creating a dialogue and relationship with the true healer, Mother Earth.

To prepare a drum for healing, rub it in a clockwise (sun direction) motion with your hand to bring your energy into it and align with it; caress it and feel its energy. Talk, sing, or chant into it, put your mouth and ear close to the drum's skin as an amplifier for your voice.

A drum healing can be used after a candle or egg reading since you have already created a map of the client's body through the diagnostics. How would you know if the client needs a drum healing? Trust your intuition. If you believe your client could benefit from it, use it. You can use your hand to play the drum to bring in more feminine energy or use the drumstick to bring in more masculine energy.

Here's how you can use drumming in a healing session:

1. The client can either be lying down or standing up.

2. Start with an energy scan of the client's body using your hands. Move from top to bottom to find areas of the body that need special attention.

3. Hold the drum by the rim while you play to stay clear of the negative energy that comes back from the client. The energy from the client must go into the drum and not be blocked by your hand. The drum should not be too big and heavy to hold.

4. Start drumming above the client's head and move down to the feet. Drum with equal strength all along the body at least four times. Watch how the body reacts.

5. Now go to the areas were you felt energy temperature fluctuations or the areas you know are energetically blocked. (Often they are the head, heart, stomach, and sexual area).

6. To extract blocked energy beat the drum over the spot and slowly increase the tempo and volume for a minute or so to let the blockage dissolve. Then lift the drum up sharply and quickly, like you're flinging the energy out to the sky, and send it away through a window or to a candle flame on your altar. Repeat at least four times for each blocked area.

7. To bring in new and good energy place the drum high above the spot you have chosen. Start drumming softly and increase the speed and power, then at once bring the drum quickly down to a few inches from the spot. Repeat at least four times for each area that needs new, good energy.

8. To conclude the session drum softly above the client's body starting from the head and move slowly down to the feet. As you go, send the lingering negative energy away to a window or candle flame in swiping motions.

SHAMANIC HEALING SUPPORT GROUP

True to many indigenous societies, meaningful and long-lasting healing can best happen when a close family or a trusted community surrounds those in need of healing with love and acceptance, witnessing the lonely and shameful battle they face. By acknowledging the struggles but also the strength and beauty of those who are suffering, the community becomes committed to the transformational process in a supportive group celebration. Charles's story below is a great example of this tradition.

He sat in the circle on the floor, a tall, thin man, twiddling his long fingers. He nervously stroked his long honey-colored hair.

"Did you see anything?" I asked Charles when it came his turn to share. "No, I saw nothing. It's stupid. I can't do it. I told you I don't see anything. It's useless." He lowered his face to meet the carpet. The single candle in the center of our circle was shining with a bright light in the dimmed room. We had just ended a shamanic journey, asking our spirit guides to show us our personal gifts and how we can manifest them in our lives.

"Did you see lines, shapes, or have any thoughts?" one of the members asked. "Not really, maybe, yeah, I saw this image of a jaguar," he admitted and looked up as if he was caught with his hand in the cookie jar. "Where was he?" she asked. "I don't know; it's stupid." "And what else?" she confronted him. "Well, I don't know. The jaguar said something; I can't remember exactly. I think he said that I needed to be proud of my gifts. Oh, I don't know; maybe I made it all up."

We all looked at each other and smiled, as that had been an ongoing theme in Charles's life, rejecting and dismissing his own gifts as an artist. Since he joined our group two years ago he had gained much confidence and grown so much that now he was now considered by many to be at the top of his profession. We waited patiently to hear what more he had to say. He was obviously battling with himself.

"OK, I'll tell you." He nervously rocked back and forth on his pillow. "I did not want to say it, but I broke my vow not to drink anymore.

I made it three years ago when I went clean and sober. I feel so shitty." He straightened up and looked at us with his sad deep hazel eyes. "OK. Now I said it." He breathed deeply and smiled in relief, looking at the group members' faces. "I admitted it. But I also want to say that I think it was a good thing."

"How?" another member asked. "It gave me such a hangover headache, I was paralyzed the next day. During that time I realized how much progress I have made since then. How much better I have become, and that is a good thing." We all agreed.

"Do you know why you took that drink?" I asked him.

"I don't know. At the end of the night somebody offered it to me. Maybe because I worked with the top person in my field and got frightened and overwhelmed," he reflected.

"Did he like your work?" someone else asked him. "Yes, yes, he even said it to my bosses too," he said proudly and laughed broadly.

"Why do you always use 'I don't know' and 'stupid'?" one of the members asked him. "I don't know; maybe I don't want to take responsibility for who I am and my gifts. I actually made a point to myself that I need to stop using those demeaning negative words," he said.

Three years earlier I had started a weekly meeting with a small group of my clients. It is one of the most amazing experiences I have had as a shamanic practitioner. It is such a blessing to see people who are committed to their inner growth and who are finding their identity and personal power and sailing forward with their lives.

Members' accomplishments have been many. One of the members went on to form his own shamanic circle and is now a teacher and a healer. Another got up the courage to ask for and receive an overdue raise and got out of his chronic debt. Another moved on to a better job she had believed prior she was not worthy of. Yet another stopped her social drinking and found love and marriage despite her prior belief that she was not made of marriage material. Some have become healers themselves and healed their family relationships. Several finished writing their books or followed their dreams in other ways. This was all thanks to the deepest support from members of the group.

At the weekly shamanic support group we use shamanic tools such as individual and partner journeys, soul retrieval, invisible cord cutting, and other ceremonies. But mainly we use the talking stick process to engage in openhearted dialogue and deep listening. The members feel safe to share their deepest fears and traumas. We learn many lessons together, mostly realizing that we are all mirrors of one another and should avoid judging one another. We've also learned that listening deeply, being supportive, and helping one another is key for personal and community growth. I often offer members homework assignments to practice during the week, which helps them be more conscious of their actions.

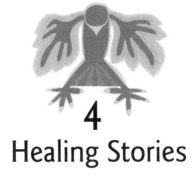

4
Healing Stories

Shamans have a health-care system in sharp contrast to our disease-care system in that they don't treat symptoms only; they use their tracking skills to find the origin of disease and treat it at its source.

ALBERTO VILLOLDO, PH.D.

The short healing stories in the following pages are all true. They were written based on my memory, notes taken after sessions, and e-mail correspondences. Believe me: I couldn't have made up those stories even if I wanted to. The names and sometimes the gender have been changed to protect my clients. Some gave me permission to use their real names. Some of the dialogue may have altered slightly.

The stories are organized according to Western categories, such as "Physical Ailments," "Anxiety," and "Depression," so that you the reader can more easily understand the processes. However in the shamanic and in many "alternative" healing modalities, we look at all diseases as energy imbalance and no distinction is made between the physical and emotional. In the shamanic tradition we do not assign labels to emotional disorders such as paranoia, schizophrenia, and depression, as we believe that doing this creates a negative social stigma. The client may wrongly identify with his disease, as in "I am schizophrenic" becomes who I am, rather than an imbalanced state that I can change. This identification can then inhibit the healing process.

My heart is full of gratitude to my clients who trusted in me, gave me the rare opportunity to peer into their most private worlds and intimate feelings, and allowed me to expand my knowledge, which I'm gratefully sharing with you in the hope it will transform your own life as well as the lives of your loved ones.

PHYSICAL AILMENTS

◈ *Broken Elbow: Dancing Again*

The undeniable cracking sounds coming from the egg in my right hand shook me out of the trancelike healing mode I was in. Before I could do anything, the egg exploded loudly. I opened my eyes. In my hand were pieces of broken shell. The bright yellow yoke and the liquid egg white were splashed all over my client's hand and were dripping down on the red, white, and blue Lakota patchwork blanket at his feet. "What a mess," I was thinking, praying my client would not notice.

I stopped. My client, sensing that something unusual had happened, opened his eyes wide and turned his head toward me. We both looked at each other in astonishment. "You know this is the elbow that broke in a car accident I had last year," he said in his soft voice, as if he was trying to comfort me. "I forgot to tell you before we started," he apologized. I grabbed some paper towels and cleaned up the mess on his hand and the blanket below.

"Close your eyes," I asked him, and I continued rubbing another egg on that wounded elbow and went on to finish his La Limpia healing ceremony. "It felt like a lightning bolt piercing through my elbow," Aaron said later, as we sat down to talk about his experience. "Let's see what happens in the next few days," I suggested.

Aaron, a tall and lanky dancer in his early forties, and also a healer himself, was curious to know why I was using eggs. "It's an old technique used in the Andes, but not only there," I told him and continued to explain how it works.

"Can I use it myself at home?" Aaron asked.

"Yes, of course you can. You can roll, rub, or vigorously shake them up and down your body to stimulate it and to release trapped energy or concentrate on special acupressure points or areas that need special attention," I told him.

"I'll try," he promised.

"Have eggs exploded while you've worked on other clients?" Aaron asked.

"Oh yes, many times," I laughed. He was curious so I went on. "One time an egg exploded on the ankle of a woman with cancer. Another exploded on a woman who had pain in the back of her neck and it splashed on her expensive white Angora top. She wasn't upset, just covered it with her black mink fur coat. And there are many more instances. But the best one was when an egg flew into the air because it had so much energy. I managed to catch it before it hit the floor. There was another time when I was working on a guy with an addiction. Whenever I rolled the eggs over his solar plexus, he screamed with pain. It took eight eggs to remove his heartache."

"Do you want to hear another story?" I asked him. "One client, an older woman in her early eighties, came to me because of severe urinary problems she was having, which improved greatly. But what was amazing was that since she was legally blind I treated her with the eggs on her eyes as well; two weeks later she came back and she claimed she started to see clearly, almost 20/20, and had started reading again."

"That is quite unbelievable," Aaron responded.

The next morning Aaron called with great enthusiasm in his voice. "You would not believe what happened; I can stretch my arm all the way. I finally have full range of motion again. It's a miracle." I was thrilled to hear the news. "I have been going to physical therapy the whole year and had some improvement, but I wasn't able to open my arm, now I can dance again." Aaron was elated.

◈ Chronic Back Pain—Yoga Instructor

I got a call from a yoga instructor: "I have had chronic back pain for twenty years. I have been to many therapists and nothing has helped. One of my yoga students told me how you healed her back pain. Can you do it for me too?" I gave her my standard answer in cases like these: "I can't promise. It's in spirit hands, but I will do my best."

On the appointed date she came in, a tall, slim, fit woman in her late sixties with a long, honey-colored ponytail. Following the diagnostic reading, I set up the massage table and asked her to lie face down. I explained that at some point in the middle of the cleansing ceremony, I would be using takuma needles—the Amazonian technique that uses the long black thorns of the takuma palm tree. "Will it hurt? Are you going to stick them in my skin like acupuncture needles?" she asked, worried.

"I will not puncture the skin. I'll only tap on it lightly with the needles. It might hurt you a bit in some places, as those are the places that need healing. I will work on your back, neck, the palms of your hands, and your feet. The needles will release tight muscles and tissues that are holding fear and traumas. Native healers use them to invigorate and stimulate the nervous system and send messages to the brain to start sending healing energy to those organs. When you feel pain, take a deep breath and release it forcefully. You can also yell, scream, or call me names if it will help," I told her. "OK, I trust you," she said hesitantly.

"Thank you," she said after the session was over. "That was interesting. It did hurt, but I'm used to pain." She laughed.

"Let me know how you are doing," I told her as she left my office. To my disappointment she never did, and I wondered from time to time if she was upset or hated the takuma needles or me. Maybe spirit failed us? Maybe I didn't do my best?

Then, two years later, the phone rang. "Hi, do you remember me?" I didn't recognize either her name or her voice. "I'm the yoga teacher. You healed my lower back. Remember? It was amazing. I was pain free for two years—no pills, nothing," she exclaimed.

"Oh, that's great. I am happy to hear that," I said, relieved. "Can I book another appointment now? The pain is back, but only slightly, just 20 percent of it, but I want you to heal that too." And so she came back for another session. That was almost two years ago; I did not hear from her again. I guess it's all good.

MARITAL PROBLEMS

◇ *Angry Red Fox*

I first met Deborah on a wintery Sunday when she stormed into my office on black-lacquered high heels. A tall, well-dressed woman from the Upper East Side, she was visibly out of her mind with anger and frustration. Her green eyes were red and bulging. Settling in the chair across from me, she brushed her fashionably cut honey-colored hair from her face and pointed in my direction with a long sharp red nail.

"I came to you because I want you to do something, you know, magic, to force my husband to give up his share of our apartment sale!" she said hysterically. "He's a jerk. I'm not going to give him his share, even though I agreed to it when we separated." She leaned over the altar, almost reaching me. "You're a shaman. I know you can do something about it." Then she straightened herself up and waited stoically.

I took a deep breath. "I'm sorry; I don't practice magic or cast spells," I answered her calmly. Her pretty face looked hurt and disappointed like a spoiled child who can't take rejection. "But we can work to see what the real problem is," I said. "Whatever you say," she said with resignation.

"Let's start with a candle and palm reading first." When I told her I could see she was holding a lot of old anger, always feeling like she was losing her personal power, and had a great need for intimacy, I could sense she was deeply touched and became more reflective.

"It's all true; I feel so lost," she finally admited.

"Would you like to have a cleansing ceremony now?" I offered, sensing that words wouldn't do much good. "OK, if that's what it takes," she said.

This story eventually ended happily, not just for her but also for the whole family. However to get there Deboarh had to go on a remarkable healing journey.

When she returned two weeks later, Deborah was a different person. "I had a very strong emotional reaction to our first session. I experienced unexplained deep sadness and uncontrollable crying. I was so emotional; it was the worst time of my life," she said as if to herself. I smiled. "Great," I said. "Now we can start to work."

Repeatedly, the issue of her tantrums and uncontrolled hysterical reactions to life's situations came up in her stories. "I know they are doing it to me to make me feel wrong, and I'm sick of it," Deborah exclaimed. "Can you give me more examples?" I asked her. She replayed a few occasions when her parents, her husband, her two daughters, people at work, and others made her become abusive and hysterical toward them.

"It's really not my fault; they are all doing it to me," she said over and over. In one case, she completely blew her top. "You see, I made a dinner reservation with my husband in an expensive restaurant. It was supposed to be our anniversary celebration. I came on time, but he didn't show up. I was so hurt. I took it as his personal statement against me. So after fifteen minutes, I stormed out of the restaurant. I'm not going to wait for that jerk. I refused to talk to him for three days."

"But, why was he late?" I asked her. "Well, there was a traffic accident, and he was stuck in it. But he could have . . ." She raised her eyes, adjusted her hair, and took a big breath.

"Oh, my God, I can now see my pattern," she exclaimed. "That is horrible, but how can I control it?" She sank into her chair with her face down and her arms hugging her body. I let her sit there for a few long minutes to contemplate what she had just admitted to herself. "Let's do a special cleansing ceremony to remove your anger first," I suggested.

As she stood in the middle of the room, I made the usual blessings ritual and closed my eyes, ready to blow her with trago. All of a sudden, an image of a red fox appeared. The animal was lying over her body. His long narrow head lay on her left breast and his body hung down around her neck as his bushy tail reached down to her knees. The fox's eyes had a glint of terror, and his face was darkened with startling rage. Through his open mouth I could see his small sharp white teeth. Maybe it is an akura, an evil spirit, or maybe it's her power animal, but why is he so angry? I thought to myself. I knew she hadn't retrieved a power animal yet, but maybe she had a special connection to a red fox.

Throughout the ceremony I kept prodding the fox's spirit to leave her energy body. I used green leaves, fire, and smoke, and finally cut his presence with my Brazilwood sword. Toward the end of the ceremony, to my amazement, I observed the fox walking slowly away with sad resignation just at her shoulder height. He walked away from her left side and slipped out through the crack under the door. As I blew the final ocarina whistle behind her neck, a thought of doubt sneaked in. Did I make it up? I needed to know.

"How do you feel?" I asked her as we sat down by my altar. "Lighter, as if a whole lot of weight lifted off me," she replied with a big grateful smile.

"Yes, it's true. I understand," I said. "And by the way, do you have a red fox as power animal?" I asked her. "No. Why do you ask?" she hurriedly replied. "Do you by any chance like red foxes?" I asked her again curiously. "Why, have you seen it?" she asked and started to laugh. "Oh, that's a long story." And she told me the story of the red fox.

"Well, many years ago my mother gave me a gift, her long black mink coat. I got tired of it a few years later and wanted something younger and more fashionable, so I traded it with my friend who gave me a beautiful red fox coat." I held my breath. "I wore it for a while and then gave it away, a few years later, to another friend. Oh, my God, I feel so guilty," she said, suddenly connecting the dots. "Is the spirit of that red fox still residing in me?" she asked, terrified.

"No, it's no longer here; it left you just now," and I went on to tell her about my vision and the spirit extraction. We sat there looking at each other in puzzlement. "Do you believe that, that spirit chose to stay with me for such a long time even though I gave it up so long ago?" she asked nervously. I shrugged my shoulders. "Maybe it had something to do with your anger as well," I said.

She collected her belongings and left quietly. A few minutes later I heard a knock on my door. I opened the door. There she was again. Her face was white as a ghost, and she was in complete distress. "What's wrong?" I asked her. She was at a loss for words. In her well-manicured hands was a winter hat made of a red fox tail. "Oh, my God, what shall

I do now?" she whispered in horror. "Well, you'll have to decide," I answered and laughed. "It was in my bag. I totally forgot about it," she said apologetically. "I think I need to let it go, and soon."

On our next session I could not believe how soft and accommodating she had become. After hearing about her progress and struggles, I asked her if she would like to journey into her future to see what would become of her. "I'm afraid to know," she honestly said. "Let's just try. If you don't like it we can always stop," I told her. I asked her to lie down on the Lakota patchwork blanket and cover her eyes. I led her on a guided journey while drumming to meet her future self, thirty years from now on another planet.

"It was amazing. I saw myself in a big beautiful house, surrounded by my husband, children, and grandchildren. It was so calm and peaceful, like a Walt Disney movie. It is probably my mind's wishes, but not necessarily the truth, right?" she asked as we sat facing each other. "It's up to you, you know," I said with a smile.

"Let's remove more stuck negative energy from you now," I suggested. She agreed, and we started the cleansing ceremony, but this time, I handed her a chonta warrior spear and asked her, with her eyes closed, to concentrate on the warrior within her.

She struggled to keep her balance and inner power. "Relax, concentrate, not with anger. Find it inside yourself and push back. Stand tall with your head up. Don't let me push you around." She did her best.

When she came back two weeks later, she was ready for a breakthrough. "How did you do it? For the past two weeks I felt much more in control, stronger, and in balance."

Drawing on the information I saw during the past candle reading, I asked her to talk about the relationship she had with her abusive father. "He always used his financial support, which I accepted, to force me to do whatever he wanted. He always treated me like an unintelligent child and kept me at his mercy. And if I did something my parents did not approve of, they would use condescending abusive language. It made me feel so helpless and angry, but I had no choice and played the obedient little girl role."

"And what about your mother?" I asked. "My mother never protected me because she feared him too. They also were not happy with my husband from the very start of our relationship, and now they don't want me to go back with him," she said in frustration.

I asked her to lie down and cover her eyes, and I led her through a guided journey in which she met her parents in the spirit world. Throughout, I encouraged her to tell them, in her mind, everything she had in her heart and was always afraid to tell them face-to-face in the real world.

"Look in their eyes. Tell them only the truth. Don't be afraid, have courage. Tell them everything you always wanted them to know about you," I pressed her. I could see she was struggling, as tears streamed down her face. I continued to drum for a few long minutes.

"Now, thank them for listening to you and change roles. Ask them to tell you whatever they never shared with you and just listen, don't answer them," I instructed her.

"How was it?" I asked her as we sat down. "I feel like I told them everything that bothered me and held inside me for so long. It felt great. They told me that they truly loved me and did whatever they believed was good for me. They said they are sorry. I am relieved and in peace. I must find ways to change the dynamics of our relationship. I must find the courage to refuse their 'gifts.' I need my independence and my self-esteem back. But tell me, how can I do that?"

"Why don't you start with their abusive phone calls?" I suggested. "When they are demanding, just let them know that this is not going to work anymore." She agreed to try.

"I was so surprised; it worked so well," she exclaimed two weeks later. "For the first time, they listened to me and allowed me to finish my sentences." And with a big smile she continued with her good news: "By the way, I also spoke to my husband; it seems that we are getting back on good terms. He is really a nice person. I don't care what my parents think of him."

Thanksgiving weekend was her biggest test. She decided to spend it with her parents, her estranged husband, and their two daughters. The visit was a triumph. Her mother for the first time let her say whatever she needed without dismissing her and actually validated her compassionately. Her father, although still somewhat dismissive, was kinder toward her, and she found herself not reacting to his words. She was happy to be with her husband. "I fell in love with him again!" she said. She made plans to move back with him. Her two daughters were very supportive as well.

Deborah was ecstatic. "What was I thinking when I first came to see you? I would like you to see my husband and one of my daughters too"—which, I did a few weeks later.

With the sale of their apartment, they bought a beautiful house in the South. "You know, I didn't need to be picky like I used to be. I found that I could surrender and be patient. And best of all, I did not have to wait thirty years for my vision to come true."

◇ Taking a Bath Together

"That's it. I want to give it a last chance," my friend Diana said to me, as she booked a healing session for herself and her husband with Don José. "Do you really want to divorce him?" I asked, surprised. "Yes. He is not responsive. I think we are finally really through."

The next Sunday, like a sacrificial lamb, her husband dragged his feet into my office with her in tow. Don José greeted them warmly and they sat down to have their candles read. It made us both feel uncomfortable listening to the bitter words they exchanged. Sometimes verbal communication can be dangerous and lead nowhere. Realizing that, Don José stopped them and asked them to take off their clothes and stand up side by side for a cleansing ceremony. Reluctantly and resentful about not having the chance to make their cases to each other they agreed.

As they stood there, breathing quietly and letting go of the frustrations, I could see their bodies started to melt away. Maybe it was Don José's chants or the oil's smell that did it, but a new expression took over their faces. After the powerful and sometimes emotional ceremony, which I assisted him with, he asked them to face each other, look into each other's eyes, and hug each other. Tears welled in my eyes. It was a miraculous moment of tenderness and acceptance. Don José looked at me, nodded in approval, and smiled mischievously. They both dressed and again took their places by the altar. This time they looked more like a couple.

"I want you to take flower baths at home," Don José told them. "Do it on Mondays, Tuesdays, and Wednesdays, before you go to sleep. Boil red and pink rose petals for ten minutes. Fill up a bucket with warm water and add the boiled petals and their water. You can also pour Agua de Florida or rose oil or any other flowery perfume into the mix. Stand facing each other in the bathtub. Then each of you will take turns pouring the water on each other: six times over the left shoulder, six times over the right shoulder, six times over the head, six times over the front, and six times on the back. Don't shower after the ceremony and don't towel dry. Just let yourselves air dry. And go to sleep." They left happy but I did not hear from her, and I wondered.

A few months later Diana called about another issue. "How's the relationship between the two of you?" I curiously and cautiously asked her. She laughed. "Couldn't be better. We are on our second honeymoon." I laughed in relief. The bath ceremony was definitely a great igniter. Don José so elegantly demonstrated again the coyote's trickster nature in his shamanic healing tradition.

◈ Singing Together

"Before I make the biggest decision of my life to marry my girlfriend, can I bring her to you so we can do a shamanic couple's session? Just to make sure we really fit. Can you do that?" my longtime friend Ohad asked me. "Sure, I've worked with many couples before. It's always very interesting. Does she agree to it?" I asked. "I'll ask her and will let you know. I'll call you later." And he hung up the phone.

And so they arrived, so much in love, admiring each other with big doe eyes. I invited them to sit around the altar. "Let's start with candle- and palm-reading divinations first, so each of you can listen in." That went quite well, as they seemed to know each other quite well. We talked openly about their personal situations, needs, characters traits, and life missions. Then I asked them to sit on the carpet face-to-face and hold hands.

"Now, each of you in turn is going to sing a love song, in which you will express to your partner how your heart feels about the other. Please keep looking into your partner's eyes throughout the singing, and make it last at least ten minutes. It doesn't have to be with words. You can just sing the melody, as long as you put your heart's intention into it."

They were surprised. They looked into each other's eyes in anticipation and finally shrugged their shoulders and agreed. "Who wants to be first?" I asked. "I'd like to go first," Dawn said. For the next ten long minutes Dawn poured her heart out to him. With tender sounds and magical words streaming out of her, she let her heart describe her love and devotion for him. At last, when it was over, Ohad's eyes were full of tears and uninhibited admiration. He reached out to her, stroked her long blond curly hair, and they hugged for a long time. "Thank you, my love," he finally said.

"I guess it's my turn now." Ohad smiled as he prepared himself. He raised his head, looked straight into Dawn's green eyes, and started to sing a beautiful ancient love song. Sweet words poured out of him with pure meaning and total gentleness. When it ended, he took a big breath and smiled at her, and they hugged again.

"Ohad, what did you feel Dawn was telling you?" I asked him. "It was amazing. She really gave herself to me. Totally with love and surrender. It was remarkable. Thank you, Dawn," he said.

"Dawn, what did you hear in Ohad's song?" I asked her. "To tell you the truth," she said, looking at Ohad sternly, "I felt like you don't know me yet. Sorry, your song was beautiful, but it was sung to some abstract female. I did not feel you were singing it to *me*." She lowered her head. There was a long moment of uncomfortable embarrassment hanging in the air. Ohad took off his heavy glasses and cleaned them. He put them back on and stroked his long beard with his hand a few times, looking at her sad face for a clue. He seemed miserable and confused by her words. "I don't know what to say," he responded.

"I think it is a time for a cleansing ceremony for both of you. I will try to clear the negative energy around and within you," I finally said to break the silence. "But, I will also try to bring new energy of love. Take off your clothes." Naked they stood side by side breathing deeply and waiting.

When they left my office after the cleansing ceremony, I wondered to myself if that union would ever take place. I wasn't sure myself what she had meant or how Ohad would react to it. But a few months later, I got a surprise.

Ohad called. "Would you like to do a shamanic ceremony to officiate our wedding?" he gingerly asked. "Really? What happened after our session?" I was curious. "It was hard to hear Dawn telling me the truth, but it was also very important. I feel we became even closer. Thank you. I am very, very happy."

As I blew Agua de Florida and threw flowers petals on them and rang the high-pitched bells during the beautiful ceremony held at the crowded Chapel of Sacred Mirrors in New York City, I kept thinking about that couple's journey and the healing power of our voices to express our truth and bring us closer.

POSSESSION

◈ *Accepting Her Faith*

The man's voice on the phone sounded deeply distraught and concerned. "My wife, Stella, is possessed. She has an entity crawling on her back. We've been to many healers, but none of them have helped her. It has ruined her and also my own life. Can you see her soon?" he begged.

Reluctantly, I agreed to see her, as a memory of another possession case was still very fresh in my mind. A young woman came to see me. All the indications were that she was truly possessed by evil spirits. The jaguar bone shook uncontrollably in her hands, the sulfur stick broke in the middle as she held it, her eyes were glazed, and all her stories confirmed it. But my spirit warned me to send her away as soon as possible.

So I proceeded with a long cleansing ceremony, and after she left, I purified my office thoroughly. I felt downright guilty, but I had to trust my guides. So this time I was hoping that it was not a possession, but I did not know what to expect.

On the day of our appointment, I opened my door to let her in. She was not alone; her concerned husband was with her. She was in her early forties, tall and slim, dark skinned, with a beautiful face with large sad dark almond-shaped eyes. She was tense and nervous. I quickly scanned her as I let them in. But they were not alone. Behind them was something I had not expected.

"You know, there are three tall, dark women, your ancestors, standing around you?" She looked surprised. "And do you know what they are saying?" I asked. "No, what are they telling you?" she asked, concerned. "They are saying that you need to do your work." "What do you mean my work?" she asked. "Become the healer you were born to be." I looked her straight in the eyes. "I don't believe it, I don't believe it, I don't believe it," she repeated, as she walked to the red couch. She sat down holding her head in her long beautiful hands. She looked up at me. "You are the third psychic to tell me this." The three spirits were now giggling with joy and satisfaction as they finally were able to bring her to me and deliver their important message.

Her husband, who was a handsome guy from Afghanistan with long curly black hair, interrupted us. "Can you remove the entity from her? She really suffers a lot. It's ruining our lives." He sounded terribly anxious.

As we sat by my altar for a candle diagnostic reading, I could see a dark energy of sadness in the flame but not the entity. So, I tested her. As she held the jaguar bone between her fingers, her hands didn't tremble even slightly, and when she held the sulfur stick, there was not even a faint cracking sound. "I believe you are not possessed," I declared to her disappointment. "Maybe these are your ancestors who are trying to get your attention and get their message to you." I was relieved that now I didn't need to perform the series of extraction ceremonies. But I could see that she did not believe me.

"But I feel its strong presence in my back. It is crawling up my left side and going up to my head. It's constantly hurting me. It's also saying different things to hurt me," she said, pointing to where the entity traveled.

I took a big breath and looked at the candle's flame again. It had a special radiance that showed me that she had spirit helpers, which surrounded and protected her. "Do you feel their presence?" I asked her carefully. "All the time," she confirmed. "Do you have visions?" "Yes." "You really are very highly connected to spirit. Let me look at your palms," I asked her.

I took a close look at her open palms under the candle's flame. "The lines on your palms say that your life is a life of service to others. You are wired to be a powerful healer. You are highly intuitive as your real power comes from the moon, the feminine home. You are passionate and have a strong need to express yourself. You could be a great writer, poet, singer, or musician. Do you do any of these things now?" I asked her. "Some, but not since this horrible intrusion happened," she said in a very low tone.

Her irritated husband shot up from his place on the couch. "Can you do something to remove it?" He was trying to hurry me up. "This thing is ruining our life and my business. Please try," he pleaded.

I heard Ipupiara's words in the back of my mind reminding me, "Sometimes even if a shaman can't see the intrusion, he must act on it." So, I reluctantly agreed to try. What ensued was worthy of a blockbuster Hollywood movie production.

First Extraction

It was late afternoon. A soft dim light came through the half-closed venetian blinds on the open windows. Stella removed her clothes and was now clad in her underwear. I invited her to lie on the red, white, and blue Lakota patchwork quilt.

I called on the three mountain spirits and those of my teachers to protect all of us in the room. I stood in the East, where everything begins, and blew trago on her and then in all the directions. Then I began to gently pound her, starting at the crown of her head, with a bunch of green leaves, which akuras (evil spirits) detest, all the while chanting my prayers. To my surprise, her body immediately started to convulse, stretching and twisting uncontrollably in all directions. A huge growl came out of her open twisted mouth. "Get out of me! You hear me! I don't want you in me! Go away! Leave me alone! What do you want from me?" she yelled in a raspy low voice, over and over again.

I kept on pounding harder. "Get it out!" I yelled, encouraging her to get rid of it. Soon it appeared her throat was blocked. A white stream of foam started dripping out of the corner of her mouth. Horrified, I was concerned that she was choking. Her husband, watching from the couch, jumped to his feet. He grabbed a few napkins and started wiping her now sweaty face and mouth while quietly reciting an ancient Afghan prayer over her body.

I kept on heavily pounding her with the green leaves, demanding that the entity leave her body right then and there. She kept stretching and twisting, her arms now above her head, while she screamed and gurgled, the foam flowing from her mouth and half choking her. Her husband was feverishly trying to wipe it as she vomited on the patchwork quilt. Now frightened, he increased the volume of his prayers, no more soft murmuring.

Now the three of us were in a total trance, chanting, praying, and screaming all at the same time. Surprised, I noticed that some part of my soul was hovering above me, watching objectively like a drone on the activity below. Strangely, I heard myself speaking and chanting in an ancient language, unknown to me. I proceeded to cover her with a new heap of green leaves and to wave thick copal smoke on her with my condor feather. The room filled with a thick cloud of smoke.

Her husband now lost all his inhibitions and hang-ups and began yelling those Afghan prayers in an unabashed fashion, while he continued to nurse her and wipe her mouth. There was no time to waste. I continued with the eggs extraction, sucking the bad spirits out of her forehead, heart center, and navel and spitting the bad energy and disposing of the eggs in a special plastic bag in the corner. Then her body seemed to relax. I covered her body from head to toe with a good amount of cornmeal and created a cornmeal circle around her, leaving a small opening allowing for the spirit intruder to leave. "Whoever you are, I command you to leave now. It is your last chance to leave!" I howled. "Do it now before I close the circle, and you will never be able to be free again." I repeated this warning to the evil spirit two more times. I took a big breath and observed her carefully as her body relaxed some more, and then I closed the circle with the rest of the cornmeal. Standing outside of the circle, I grabbed some sea salt and rubbed her body from head to toe to remove the leftover entity. She was now exhausted but at peace. I stepped aside and blew Agua de Florida from all sides over her and covered her with red and white carnations, to fill in the void the departed entity's energy left.

Her husband was now quiet at his place on the couch, watching over the procedure. I removed the flowers and continued to close the energy field and protected her with my black healing stones. She was breathing normally. I laid one clear quartz crystal on her third eye to clear and balance her spiritual energy and one purple amethyst on her heart to safeguard her from psychic attacks and moved away, letting her rest. I watched her as she quieted down, her body now completely relaxed. She almost fell asleep. She was drained, and so was I.

"What was that all about?" she asked me as she sat in front of me at the end of the ceremony a few minutes later. "You did very well. You pushed it almost all the way out," I assured her. "We need to do two more ceremonies soon to get rid of it entirely."

"Not all of it? Can you remove it completely?" her husband asked in fear. "I can only try to do my best," I answered. "Would it be the same ceremony?" he asked nervously. "No, it will be a stronger one. Get ready." He was worried after seeing what had happened before. Stella tied back her headscarf, raised her head, looked me in the eyes, and said, "My spirit guides told me I should trust you. I will be back." I was glad to hear a new willpower in her voice.

Second Extraction

A couple of days later, we were sitting around the altar again. "I feel somewhat better, but I still feel that energy crawling on my back and into my head," she said. When I raised the issue of sexual abuse, she confided in me that she had been abused as a young girl. She lowered her eyes and said, "I never fully resolved it. My narcissistic and powerful mother, who barely raised me and gave me away to my grandma, is a world-famous healer and spiritualist in our community in the Caribbean Islands. She recognized my talents at a very young age but did not want me to compete with her." From his seat on the couch her husband interjected, "Stella is a great musician and had an impressive international singing career until this entity took over her life." I thanked him for the information. "Now I'm helping my husband in his design business," she said quietly.

This time the ceremony started in much the same way, except now all the players immediately lost any embarrassment they may have had. Stella was more assertive with her attached spirit. Her husband continued helping her, in a loud voice encouraging the spirit to leave while he wiped her mouth like an experienced nurse.

Toward the end I took a round red mirror off the wall and placed it in front of her face, as Ipupiara once taught me. I instructed her to open her eyes. "Look into the mirror. Do you see the intruding spirit?" Slowly she opened her beautiful eyes. I could see the frozen horror in them. "Yes, I do!" she murmured, and her body shivered. "Look him in the eyes and tell him to leave you now!"

There was no force in the world that could stop her screaming, yelling, and crying now. "Get out of me! You hear me! I don't want you in me! Go away! Leave me alone!" She demanded, begged, and ordered the entity with a deep raspy voice. Her faithful husband stood by, wiping the gushing white foam that poured from her mouth. It took a few more minutes, and her body relaxed. She closed her eyes.

I then finished the ceremony with tobacco smoke, covered her with red and white carnations, and went on to create a protection ring around her with the black stones. All the while Stella rested quietly, exhausted, lying under a bunch of crystals and a pile of fresh green leaves. This time they left quietly, no words needed to be said, taking in the powerful ceremony.

Third Extraction

A few days later, we proceeded with a different kind of ceremony. Stella already felt stronger and even smiled broadly for the first time. Still she felt the energy presence on her back. "But I don't pay much attention to it," she said.

"So when are you starting your healing practice?" I asked her. "I am going to do it. I promise," she assured me. "Remember those three women ancestors. They will not rest until you do," I warned her.

In our final ceremony, the atmosphere was much more relaxed. It lacked the drama of the first two. During the cleansing ceremony I concentrated on removing and detaching the remnant of dark energy that was still attached to her. It was hard to believe she was the same person who first came to my office.

"I think you need to do a cord-cutting ceremony," I proposed. "What's that?" she asked, worried. I explained that in this ceremony she would be able to pull out and detach the emotional hooks her mother and the entity attacker had placed in her. "What do you mean by emotional hooks?" She was curious. "When people hurt and abuse us either emotionally or physically, that energy is stored in our body's tissues and then in our organs. We need to sever those ties to them so that they lose their power over us and we are set free to live our own lives. Otherwise, we become their puppets, and they can pull our strings," I explained. She nodded her head and agreed.

Again, she lay down, and I started to drum. In a few short minutes her long thin hands where busy moving up and down and sideways, forcefully pulling out invisible filaments from all parts of her body. When she was completely done, I stopped drumming. "I feel clean and free," she said. "Thank you. It was very powerful."

As we sat for our final consultation, we brought new clarity to the issues she was dealing with and planned her next life moves. She was sitting up tall, quite confident, and even smiling. She did not feel like a client anymore, more like a powerful colleague.

Her husband, on the other hand, was seemingly now agitated. "I think you need to have your own session," Stella calmly told him. And so he did the next week. I met them once more in a solstice ceremony I held. They looked relaxed and content. "We are doing well," she whispered before they left.

◇ Dark Entity

Dear Mr. Beery,

I would like to know if you believe you would be able to assist me. In October 2013, I believe a dark entity attached itself to me and has since that time orchestrated an extremely wide array of previously unencountered and bizarre effects and sensations upon me. The majority of these involve the infliction of pain and discomfort through the apparent use of "rays" and "waves" directed to a body part, particularly the genitalia. This infliction has escalated to a point that could be described as almost continuous torment and torture. The sensations also include the perception that the entity is almost constantly above me, or inside my physical body, at any location. The objective of this torment and torture is intimated to be my personal destruction. I have consulted internists, dermatologists, urologists, psychiatrists, and a neurologist regarding the unexplained sensations and associated pains, but no specialist in any of these fields has found any pathology. I believe that I require soul retrieval and an entity extraction.

So read the e-mail I received one day.

"Should I tell you why I'm here?" the man asked with a soft British accent as he sat down by my altar. I could see the fear in his eyes. I took a look at this well-dressed, tan, and handsome man in his midforties. "No, it is not necessary. Let me do a candle reading, and we'll see what happens."

He took off his clothes, closed his eyes, and, concentrating, passed the white candle over his entire body. Sitting by the altar I chanted to connect to my spirit helpers for protection and assistance. When he finished, as instructed he blew three times on the candle and handed it to me. I lit the flame and took a look.

"It seems like you are very well connected to spirit. Probably having visions and dreams," I said. "I'm not spiritual. I don't meditate, and I don't remember my dreams," he curtly replied. "But you have no faith. You have a huge black cloud of fear located in your stomach and around your heart," I continued. "That's true. I have digestive problems, since that thing started." "You also have a pattern of repeating dark negative thoughts." "Yes, that's true too," he agreed. "I can see that you believe or have had experience with aliens?" He looked surprised. "I didn't believe in aliens before this all happened, but now I do. This entity comes from above and sucks energy from my stomach," he said, pain evident in his voice.

"Inside the candle's flame by the wick I can see a man figure with dark skin. He is tall and thin and has very short black hair. Is that person your previous relationship?" I asked him. I could see he was uncomfortable. "No, I don't recall anyone like that," he said. "Did you have a sexual relationship with him when this thing started?" I pressed on. He twisted in the chair and took a deep breath. "Oh, I think I know who you are talking about." His face had darkened. "Who is he?" I asked. "I was experimenting with crystal meth at that time. He was my dealer, and yes, we had sex a few times, but we only fooled around," he said. "Can I ask you an intimate question? Did you allow him to penetrate you?" He blushed and leaned back on his chair, took a minute, and then said, "Yes, I did. I don't know why. I usually don't do that. I am a top. But this time I went on with it, and it felt very good to surrender to him. We were not really in a relationship," he said quietly, and then he jolted. "You mean to tell me that the entity could be him?" he asked, surprised. "I don't know yet, but something must have happened between the two of you that made him very envious and jealous of you. Can you think why?" I asked, while I looked at the candle, trying to find the answer myself. "No, why would he do it?" I pressed on: "Did you do something that could have made him jealous?" He took a minute to think about it. "You may be right; I think I might have." His face became pale. "He introduced me to his friend who also sold crystal meth, and we hit it off. We became sexual partners. He wasn't happy about that. . . . Oh, my God, do you think he did it?" he gasped. "Well, he might have," I said. "Is he from the Dominican Republic?" I asked, as I got new information from the flame. "Yes, he is. How do you know that?" He was startled. I went on, "He probably asked someone else, a woman, to do the curses to inflict the pain on your genitals. Do you understand now why he did it?" I could see him processing this new information, and a great discomfort spread throughout his lean body.

At that moment I remembered a similar case many years ago in which an angry and jealous spirit, an aunt of my client, sent curses from the other side to physically hurt him in his groin. She insisted on taking revenge on his mother, her hated sister, by causing this middle-aged man extreme pain. It got so bad that he could hardly walk. When I relayed this information to my client, he confirmed my physical and emotional description of his aunt. He said that she never married, had no children of her own, and was bitter and jealous of his successful mother. It took lots of effort and threats during a few sessions to convince her to release him and remove her sharp claws out of his private parts.

"Let me look at your palms." He moved forward and opened his palms. "You have healer lines, many of them. You also have strong lines of intuition. You are extremely stubborn and very independent. Although you desire intimate relationships, you are very careful and don't have much trust in your partners." He looked surprised. "I am not spiritual, and I'm not a healer. I am a very practical and logical man. I am a lawyer," he said proudly. I continued my reading: "Your fingers indicate that your emotions are easily manipulated by logic, probably by your mother." "That's true," he confirmed, "but lately we have a better relationship." "To be a healer you don't have to do what I do," I told him. "Let me ask you, when you have sex, do you take special care of your partners and make sure they enjoy themselves and are satisfied?"

"Oh yes. I'm very proud of that," he said. "As a lawyer do you make sure your clients are dealt with fairly and are always satisfied?" I asked him. "Yes, it's true. I see the connection you are making. I never thought about it in this way."

"Okay, are you ready to do the cleansing and extraction ceremony now?" I asked him. "Yes, I would love that." He undressed and stood at the center of the room and I went to work. I handed him two sulfur sticks to hold in both hands. "The sticks will draw any evil and negative energy from your body," I told him. I called on the mountains and my teachers' spirits for help, and just before I closed my eyes, I noticed hovering above his left shoulder a malicious dark entity. I forcefully blew trago from all four directions at the affected areas on his body, and then I struck and cleared him with the branches of green leaves, urgently removing that entity from above his shoulder. He startled and started sobbing. Next, I pounded on my drum to shake any stalled energy still in his body. I took the green branches, blew Bacardi 151 on them, lit them on fire, and strongly tapped the blue flames on his bare skin. Then I spread heavy copal smoke all around him, especially above his left shoulder. I waited for the heavy smoke to clear and went to his head to rub and shake eggs on his entire naked body. Then I placed the eggs on a few points of his body and sucked the curse's energy out of him. As if by magic his body relaxed. I took two sharp takuma needles and poked him vigorously on his lower back and shoulder blades and behind his neck to release stuck energies of fear. His skin was now covered with heavy sweat; toxins were pouring out of him. He took a few deep breaths and released a few screams—as best as an English gentleman can do—as his body twisted in pain. I rushed to open the door wide, and with the condor feather I cleared the intruder energy out the door. When it was all over, I blew Agua de Florida and brushed him with red and white carnations to fill in the misplaced energy with new harmonious energy. His body was now relaxed, and I could continue to seal his physical and energy bodies with my volcanic healing stones for protection from further intrusion. I handed him the chonta spear and instructed him to hold it forcefully against my constant pushing. "Stand tall. Find your balance. Feel your inner power. Protect yourself from future intrusions," I instructed him. His body transformed in front of my eyes. Every muscle was now invigorated by a newfound power and determination. I blew tobacco on his hands and all over him for blessings. Then I pointed the spear to the crown of his head, heart, and below the belly button, while blowing tobacco smoke. I stood behind him, and using the tiny ceramic ocarina, I blew a sharp tune to call his soul back. I took a few steps back. The malicious black energy was not there. I poured Agua de Florida in the palm of his hands and instructed him to rub it in vigorously, starting at the top of his head and going all the way down to his legs.

"You can open your eyes now," I told him quietly. He opened his blue eyes and looked at me in a daze. "Can I give you a hug?" I asked him. "Yes, sure." But I felt his hug was hesitant, not letting himself be fully embraced.

"How did you know to suck the energy from the parts of my body where I suffered most?" he asked later as we sat down. "Well, that is why we did the candle reading first," I replied and smiled. "How do you feel?" I asked him. "Relaxed, clear, like something lifted out of me. It is strange."

I instructed him with the traditional restrictions to do after the ceremony—to sage his home and take sea-salt baths. Then I asked him to blow the candle flame away with a prayer. "You know, sometimes spirit forces us to do what we came here to do. You can look at this incident you just had as a lesson. In other words, you might have brought it on yourself to be connected to your life purpose as a healer and to faith," I said. I could see he was struggling to accept what I was saying. "In cases like yours, if you feel that the entities are coming back, we will need to perform two more ceremonies soon," I told him before he left. He did not come back.

CANCER

◈ Missing a Piece of the Puzzle

Sometime a request by a new client can be surprising. "I don't expect you to cure me. I know I am dying. I don't have much time left. I want to come for a long session, as long as it takes. I want to find out what is the source of the deep anger in me before I leave this world. I don't want to take it with me." Brenda, a woman from out of state, was telling me this on the phone. I thought she was brave, and I was looking forward to meeting her.

We agreed she would come for the following weekend. I cleared my schedule to give her the time she needed. As we sat by my altar, she softly said, "I'm an energy healer myself. Actually I have a very busy healing center down in my town. I'm quite well known in my state." I admired the directness and honesty of this well-presented woman in her midfifties.

Throughout the weekend we did diagnostic readings, and we journeyed with her power animals and spirit guides. It was when we did soul retrievals that she found that missing piece. As we sat facing each other on the blanket, she reflected, "I always suspected it was somehow connected to my mother, but I could not put my finger on it. Now I know." She sighed deeply and quietly contemplated the new information for a long while. "Would you want to try to forgive her and maybe yourself?" I suggested. "Yes, I guess that will be the last thing I need to do." She was eager to do it.

I asked her to lie down on my Lakota patchwork blanket and cover her eyes. Sitting by her side, I started with soft but fast drumbeats. Then I led her in a guided journey to meet her mother's spirit in a large clearing of a jungle beyond a river. As they saw each other, I encouraged her to invite her mother to face her, look her in the eyes, and convey to her mother everything she had never told her mother or was afraid to reveal to her—just the brutal truth, as hurtful as it may be. "Say it all; don't leave anything unsaid," I ordered her. After long minutes I asked her to reverse roles and listen to her mother telling her the same. She wept, releasing old wounds, letting them go. I stopped drumming.

"It was a very powerful meeting. I feel I am in peace now. Thank you for allowing me to piece that puzzle together. I hope I can see you again if I feel strong enough." We both knew it wouldn't happen. That was the first and last time we met. Trusting me to complete her beautiful life puzzle was a true gift.

◇ Easy Walk

It is hard to believe or explain how an immobile person can get up and walk as if she has received a shot of energy after a shamanic healing. The walking cane left in my office behind the couch reminds me every day of this story.

"My mother is very old. She has advanced cancer, stage four, and I believe you can help her. You do La Limpia, right? You have to know that she is hardly moving." So said a nice Spanish-speaking young woman on the phone that summer day.

At the appointed Sunday, the two showed up, a bit late. "I apologize. It was hard to find a taxi," the daughter said, as they slowly walked into my office. I invited the mother to sit by my altar. Her legs were heavy and swollen; she seemed extremely exhausted and lethargic from the trip, like she wasn't even sure why she was here. "I believe nothing can help me," she finally and quietly said. "There are always miracles, you never know," I told her. She did not buy it.

With the daughter acting as translator, I asked the mother to rub the candle over her body. I took a look at the flame. It was easy to see the concentrated negative energy in her belly and how it was now spreading in her body. There was no way she could stand up for the cleansing ceremony so I asked her to stay in her chair. I sprayed her with trago, cleaned her with the green leaves, smoked her with copal, and while working with the eggs, I paid special attention to the area where the flame indicated there was cancer and sucked that bad energy through the eggs, spitting it out into the waiting plastic bag. We finished with blowing Agua de Florida and sprinkling flowers for protection. As we finished I thanked her. "Gracias," she responded, a small smile cracking her face. Her eyes now were brighter, glowing as if she had just woken up from a bad dream.

"How do you feel now?" I asked her after the ceremony. "Lighter. I feel good. Thank you." And they left.

As they closed the door behind them, I looked through the window at the blue sky. I doubted the ceremony would work for her. She was too fragile and too far gone in her cancer. But then I remembered a story Ipupiara once told me, and I gained faith. "One day I was invited to perform a ceremony for a cancer patient in a hospital. I told my wife that I didn't want to go. I am not such a powerful shaman that I can cure cancer. She looked at me in surprise and said, 'Aren't you the one telling your students that it is not you who performs the healing? You tell them that it is Mother Earth and spirit who does that, isn't it? You must go.' I recognized that I did not have faith. I decided to go and be a channel to spirit, and whatever happens needs to happen. And it worked. The woman felt much better and responded better to the hospital treatment." Ipupiara's experience calmed my doubts.

The next day I received a call from her daughter. She was excited, "You would not believe what happened. When we went downstairs, I told my mother to wait by the door so I could go and look for a taxi. She refused. She said she wanted to walk home by herself—imagine, sixteen long blocks! I did not want to tell her no. So we started to walk home. She had so much energy; every block I asked her if she was okay, and she kept walking until we got to her home. It was a real miracle. When we got home she was still energized. Thank you."

EMOTIONAL BLOCKAGES

◈ *The Gatekeeper*

"I am here," said the tall broad lawyer with big piercing blue eyes, "because I want to open my heart. I'm divorced with three grown-up kids. I just came back from Peru where I participated in ayahusca ceremonies. During the *dieta,* sitting in my isolated hut by myself for ten days, fasting almost the entire time and drinking the plant medicine daily, I realized that my heart is closed and that is the reason I can't get into real satisfying relationships. I am dating a lot; I'm on a few dating sites, but nothing has really worked." Brandon went on: "Can you tell me what's wrong with me?" He looked in my eyes as if I was his last hope.

I asked Brandon to rub a candle over his body and concentrate on all the things that blocked him. I took a look at all the negative energy he was holding inside and around him. Big fear and low self-esteem popped into my head. I then took a look at his palms. "You are a stubborn man," I said. "Independent, don't like people to tell you what to do. But you are also a very sensitive, intuitive healer." "Me, a healer? You must be kidding me," he said. "Let me show you." And I showed him the lines on his hands that indicated his capacity to be a healer: "Here, seven lines under your pinky." "I never thought of myself as a healer," Brandon said puzzled.

"What happens when you meet a new woman? Do you try to understand and help her with your advice?" "Yes, I do." "Do they appreciate it?" "Not always," he said chuckling. "Did you ever wonder why you chose to become a lawyer. It's to help people, right?" He took some time to digest that. "Yes, you are right. I go above and beyond to help my clients. Interesting. I never looked at that this way." "Let's do a cleansing ceremony. I will concentrate on your heart. When you feel it, let it open."

"Many things have changed since I saw you two weeks ago. Generally, I feel I am more aware. I feel more calm and openhearted," he said during our next session. "Let's try something. Close your eyes," I told Brandon.

I asked him to put his left hand over his heart and tell me what he saw. At first he saw only complete darkness, but I kept prodding him to go deeper. He next saw geometrical shapes, lines, and triangles moving in all directions and then a ball of light on the edge of the darkness. Finally, he saw a snake with a big head, long body, and sharp piercing eyes.

"Can you ask him what he is doing there?" I asked. "He said he is protecting my heart from being hurt," he replied. "How long has he been there?" I asked. "Many years. Maybe from childhood."

I asked him if he still needed the snake and if he would be willing to let the snake go. He said yes, so I suggested that he ask the snake to leave. "The snake refused. He said no. He feels comfortable there. He said I need him," Brandon reported. "I would like him to leave. But it feels like I need faith or courage. I have to jump from the edge of the cliff. It's scary. If he leaves, where will he go?" He clearly felt anxious about abandoning the snake and its protection.

"Wherever he needs to be," I told him. "Maybe into the ether." "It's scary, but I'll try. . . . Yes. I see him disappearing."

"How do you feel now?" I asked him. "Lighter, but a bit shaky," he said.

I asked him to bring back the ball of light. He did and reported that it was no longer pitch black; it was gray. "Go deeper," I prodded him. "What do you see?"

"I see a dark silhouette of a young man. It's me. I can recognize myself," he reported. "Is he happy? Do you like him?" "Not really," he replied.

I encouraged him to go deeper still. He saw the silhouettes of a group of men. "Do you know them?" I asked. "What are they doing there?"

"They are here to initiate me. They are accepting me. I don't know who they are. But I feel really good. Happy."

Once again I prodded him to go deeper. This time he saw himself as a five-year-old. I asked him to look into the eyes of his five-year-old self and ask if he is happy. "No. I'm sad because I'm alone." "Ask your young self what he needs," I said.

"He needs somebody to love him give him affection and recognition." He promised his young self to give him what he needs. "Can you ask that boy if he would like to merge with you and enter your heart?" I asked him. "Yes. He does," he said. "Do you want to have him back?" I asked him. "Yes, very much," he replied without hesitation. "Go ahead and put your hand on your heart and allow that merging to happen." I instructed him. He lay his big hands on his heart, and after a second a big, gentle smile came across his face.

"How does it feel?" I asked. "My heart feels really warm, relaxed. No fear. Calm. Thank you."

"You can open your eyes now," I suggested. "How do you feel now?" "Vulnerable," he said. "But it feels good. I understand."

◇ Open My Heart

John stood there contemplating, talking quietly to himself. "That is really what I want. To feel like I am hugged by the world," he said as tears filled his eyes. I could feel his big heavy body trembling like a mountain before an eruption. His strong arms clutched my body tightly, in a big bear hug. We stood there for a few more minutes in the middle of the room at the end of the cleansing ceremony, breathing together, feeling the energy of our bodies and our heartbeats. "Yes, that is what I really want," he said, admitting this to himself, maybe for the first time, as he let go.

"Do you want another hug?" I asked him quietly. "Yes, please," John whispered. Savoring the magical moment we stood there together, embracing strongly, and we let our bodies melt. I read somewhere that when we embrace for twenty seconds or more, the body is able to produce a love hormone (oxytocin) that helps us relax and feel safe and quiets our fears and anxiety.

"Maybe that is what my mother meant when she told me to open my heart wide," he said, as he dressed and gathered his belongings to leave. It was not the first time I have worked with John. His mother, a client of mine, sent him to see me a year before cancer took her away. With an abusive and estranged father and distant brother he normally felt like a loser: alone, lonely, resentful, and angry. His soul was yearning for acceptance, family, and love.

As he reached the door, he stopped, turned back to look at me, and said, "I think I never let people into my heart, or get too close to me. I reject everyone. It was always me against them. I never felt I belonged." I admired his clarity and brave honesty.

I watched this lone wolf, this big, strong, heavy man, a talented musician in his midthirties, and saw his usually severe face become vulnerable childlike and lovable.

◇ The Price of Success

As she put back on her elegant business suit, Robin, a top business executive, turned around at the end of one of her sessions and said, "That was amazing. Thank you. I want to give my boss a fiftieth birthday present. He always spoke about wanting to meet a shaman. Can I gift him two sessions with you?" "Sure, why not," I replied. And that is how Joshua appeared one afternoon at my doorstep. He truly looked out of place in my healing room with his trim body, sharp business attire, perfectly trimmed blond hair, and aura of big business authority. As we sat down I glanced out the window and saw his private driver waiting on the street. It was a bit intimidating, I must confess.

"You're not from New York; where are you from?" I asked him, as I looked at his candle flame. "No, I'm a New Yorker. I've lived in New York more than twenty-five years," he said politely but as if he was challenging me. "It seems that you come from the middle of the country. I see green fields and open space, like a farm?" I went on reading. "Yes, that's true. I was raised in rural North Carolina, in a small family farm. How do you see that?" He was surprised. "I just do."

I laughed and went on looking at the flame again. "You are also deeply sad and very fearful. It looks like you are still in a fetal position in a womb, unable to open yourself up to become yourself." He looked up. His blue eyes met mine. He was truly sad and startled, as if he could not believe that someone could see his real self behind his well-constructed mask. "You feel alone and very lonely, don't you?" I pressed him. "In all honesty, yes, that's the way I feel. But no one knows. Everyone thinks I am the most happy, popular, and lucky man alive." He shook his head and smiled. "I am considered a meteoric success story, like Steve Jobs. I have everything a man can ever dream of. People admire me; they all want my company. I make my company a shitload of money and for myself too. Everything I touch becomes successful, even though I never knew what I wanted to become. It seems there is a force of success behind me. And yet I feel alone and at times lonely. I always keep myself calm and smile to everyone; that's my secret. I never get angry; I bury it well inside myself," he told me in his well-mannered voice. "I married my college sweetheart. We have two teenage girls, and we live in a prestigious neighborhood not too far from the city. I am in charge of many thousands of people all around the world. I work for one of the largest financial groups in the U.S."

"Do you have other siblings?" I asked, as I saw two of them in the flame. "Yes, in a way, because I was adopted at birth. I don't know my biological mother, who gave me up. My parents, three years later, adopted another boy and then a girl. I love my adopted parents very much." "Do you know who your biological mother is?" I asked. "I always thought about my birth mother but never wanted to find out who she was and why she gave me up. I did not want to hurt my adopted mother. Maybe I will look for her after my adopted mother is gone," he said, as if debating with himself. "I was always the best in school and in sports. I have this magical intuition to always be in the right place at the right time," he continued, quite proud of himself, and started drifting in thoughts.

"Would you like to do a cleansing ceremony now?" I suggested. "Yes, sure, let's do it." He carefully undressed and neatly folded his clothes on the couch. As the ceremony progressed, I could tell his body, muscles, and face were loosening and relaxing. He was not protecting himself anymore, and as we finally hugged, I could feel him let go; his body fully surrendered. We sat down; his face changed—no more fake smiles to make me feel good. "Thank you. I'll be back," he said, and he rushed to be chauffeured to an important event out of town.

Two weeks later he was back. "These two weeks were unexpected. So much happened," he said. "Great, tell me what happened," I asked. "It was the first time after many years that I let myself dream and just disappear in my thoughts, although it happened only on three occasions. It was so refreshing. I was also very angry." He lowered his voice as if he was ashamed. "Wonderful," I said. "What do you mean?" He was confused. "Who were you angry at?" I asked. "At my wife." "What did she say or do to you?" I went on, inquiring. "It was about something really stupid, but I let myself go, showing her my frustrations. We ended up not speaking for a whole two days. But the most surprising thing for me was that she called me at my office and thanked me for showing up and for being vulnerable for the first time in our marriage. We had three days of real closeness. Is that what happens after your ceremony?"

he asked. "Many times, to many people. This is excellent. You let your feelings flow without trying to control them. You unblocked the river, so to speak," I said. "So what should we do today?" he eagerly asked.

"Last time in the candle I saw you as a four-year-old. Do you have a picture in your mind of that time?" I asked him. "Hmmm . . . let me concentrate. Yes, I do." "Okay. Now close your eyes and bring that image up." We did a sort of soul retrieval process for his four-year-old self. He found him and learned to love and like him. The boy asked to be loved by him and play with him. He did it in his mind, and then he swore to adopt and protect him as he brought him into his heart. "That was so powerful," he said and smiled.

"Why don't we do a shamanic journey to find your power animal," I suggested. "Okay, how is it done?"

His power animal was an eagle. "It feels just like me. What does that mean?" he asked. "The eagle symbolizes your need of trust, to be able to fly in the unseen world—the air. It symbolizes not concentrating on the little details of life, to instead have a grand perspective and look for opportunities below and swiftly take them." He thought about it for a minute. "Oh, that is me; this is what I do." He was obviously pleased.

"Now let's do one more journey and ask your eagle a question, something like 'How can I heal that four-year-old boy?' Is that Okay?"

When he came back from the journey, he said, "I realized that as a child I had to be the best so that my adopted parents would justify adopting me. I always needed to be in full control, to not make any mistakes. I made myself indispensable to everyone around me to justify my existence. I became the supporter of the family. Like two bookends that hold everyone inside, I was afraid to let go because all the books would fall down from the bookshelves and disappear. On the inside I was always alone and lonely, but no one could tell because on the outside I was always smiling, positive, and supportive."

We hugged, said good-bye, and he ran downstairs for the waiting car to be driven to a very important social function he and his wife were hosting. I heard that he retired from his executive position and decided to devote himself to helping his community and other social causes.

DEPRESSION

◇ *Face in the Dirt*

It was a couple of years after we started working together that I felt Paula was emotionally ready for soul retrieval. When she first came to see me, this tall, strong woman sporting straight blond hair wanted to rid herself of unexplained deep depression, an unsatisfying profession, insecurity, and a pattern of breakups in her relationships where she gave her power away to her partners. A successful graphic designer, she was not feeling successful and continually felt powerless and overridden by her bosses. Over the time we had worked together, she had become happier and more balanced, and so I felt it was time to deal with her deeper traumas. She agreed.

Paula lay down on my Native American patchwork blanket and closed her eyes. I started drumming quietly sitting by her side, my knee slightly touching her arm. I called my spirit guide. When he appeared behind the bushes, I greeted him and explained the task in hand before me. In a split second I was taken to a countryside farm. I saw a dirty wooden fence. My eyes continued to wander; I wanted to see more. I realized it was a small cowshed. Inside there were two girls. It was young Paula, three or four years old, and an older aggressive girl. "Could it be her sister?" I asked myself. The older girl was almost boylike with shoulder-length dirty blond hair. She forcefully wrestled Paula into the mud, holding her face down in the dirt with her feet. It was hard for Paula to breathe; she felt she was suffocating and felt extreme fear.

My body shook. I felt the shock and terror the young girl was experiencing throughout my own body. Immediately, I reminded myself of the role I was playing, and I called my power animal for help and strength. I asked it to take me to the young girl's soul part she had let go of. My eyes drifted to the top of a large tree near the farmhouse. There I saw little Paula huddling in a bird nest, sheltered by soft gray feathers. She was frightened and shivering. I noticed that on her forehead was a big spot of blood. I introduced myself and asked her to come with me and return to Paula, who is now in her midthirties. "No," she refused.

"Paula herself asked me to bring you back, and she promised to take care and protect you to the best of her abilities," I told her. She wasn't sure. "My own sister that I loved and admired so much treated me in this way. How can I trust anyone else?" she protested. "Today Paula is a different person and is capable of protecting you," I reassured her. "Paula needs you now. She wants to live a happier, more fulfilling life and only you can help her," I told her. We went back and forth.

At last she agreed. I stopped drumming, put down the drum, scooped her soul part in the palms of my hands, and blew it into Paula's heart in three strong blows. Then I helped Paula sit up and blew it again three times into the crown of her head.

We sat facing each other in quietness for a few long minutes. Doubting myself, I was wondering if the event I had witnessed had any truth to it. I took a big breath and shared it with Paula.

Paula looked in my eyes with a long sad face. Tears streamed down her cheeks. Slowly she opened up to confirm that incident in her childhood. "We grew up on a farm, raising a few cows and animals. I remember that tree you saw by the house. I vividly remember my sister pushing my head to the ground and the blood flowing down my forehead. I was so scared. I was sure I was going to die. My sister was cruel to me throughout my entire childhood," she said quietly. "Did she take away my soul part?" Paula asked after a long silence. "No, you let go of it, from the abuse and humiliation and fear of death. You needed to protect yourself, which is a good thing, as you could not at that age handle it any other way," I explained. She nodded in agreement. "I hope I could handle it differently now," she said boldly and smiled.

"I think it is time to welcome the returning soul part and to integrate it back into your life. Let's do another journey," I suggested, and we went on another shamanic journey. This time she journeyed on her own. "She is so sweet and fragile. She wants me to be strong and stand up for myself," Paula shared after with glowing eyes. "I promised I would be the best mommy to her," she continued. "I would like to give you some homework to do," I said. "I want you to make or buy a small doll in the image of your three-year-old self and for the next two weeks be with her continuously. Take her everywhere you go. Eat, sleep, bathe, and work with her. From time to time ask her how she is doing and if she feels loved, safe, and proud of you." I looked at her blue eyes to see a big surprise. "Okay. I'll do it. I promise," she said with a big laugh.

Paula returned a few weeks later a different person. "How are you doing?" I asked her as we sat behind the altar. "I feel much better, even optimistic. It is so strange; I actually like my job now and have even been given more responsibilities. I am in charge of a small group of designers. I can't say that my relationship with my sister has improved— I don't expect it to—but I'm not afraid of her anymore. Even my relationship with my partner took a turn. I don't submit to her like I used to." I gave her a high five and we laughed.

◈ Dog Walker

"I want you to see my son George too. He is very depressed. I don't know what to do with him anymore. He sits in the apartment all day long, in his closed room, sleeping till late, and does nothing but eat. He has gained so much weight. I don't recognize him," a client told me, after one of our sessions.

When he came, I could see in the candle that a dark cloud of negative energy surrounded him, that he felt depressed and powerless. "Tell me, what is it that you want to do with your life?" I asked him. "I don't know," he said, unsure. "What is your dream?" I pushed on. "I want to work as a political consultant. I went to college in the Midwest to study political science. I had good times and many friends, but since I came back home and am living with my parents it seems I got lost. There are no jobs; believe me, I've been looking. I lost my dream. I gave it up. I have no friends and no relationships." He was twenty-three years old with no future.

I looked at the candle flame as it reflected on the smooth healing stone surface and saw a small white dog. "Do you have a dog at home?" I asked. "Yes." "Do you like him?" "I do like him. He's my only friend."

"Can I take a look at your palms?" I asked. "You are a strong-willed person, independent, with a strong need to help others. You also full of passion and desire intimacy." "Yes, it's true, but I don't seem to manifest it," he sadly said.

After the cleansing ceremony, when he was relaxed, I felt he started to trust me. I told him of the dietary instructions and said, "I want to give you homework. Would you mind?" "Depends what it is," he said hesitantly. "Well, from tomorrow, you will take charge of the family dog. Take him early in the morning and evening for a walk in the park near you. Can you do that?" "I guess," he said reluctantly. I don't think he understood why.

Two weeks later, I saw a changed person. Life had returned. He was relaxed and had a big smile on his handsome face. "How was it to take care of your dog?" I asked him, as we sat down. "He is a handful. I have to get up early, but it's fun," he said with a laugh. Fresh air, a daily walk in nature, and taking care of another being can do the trick.

"What should we do today?" he asked. "Well, do you want to have a power animal guide to help you in your life?" I asked him. "What is it?" he suspiciously asked. I explained the idea behind it and how the journey is done, and we did a journey. He found a teacher. "Would you like now to ask your power animal what is it that you can do to find the job of your life?" "I'll give it a try."

When he came back from the journey he had a few answers. "Are you willing to do what your power animal told you?" "Yes, I'll try." "Let's do a cleansing ceremony now. Concentrate on your inner power," I suggested.

"Will you give me homework today?" he asked before he left. "Sure, keep walking the dog, do a journey with your power animal every night before you go to bed, and do what he tells you to do."

"I have a job interview with a city councilman at the end of the week," he said, as he sat in front of me at the next session. "It's only a paid internship, but it's a start." He smiled broadly. "I also wanted to tell you that last night when I was on the train, I noticed a girl looking at me. For the first time, I smiled back at her. It wasn't much, but it felt so good."

George got the job. In a few months it turned into a regular job.

"It's very demanding, but I love it. I help so many people with their complaints, trying to help them with the city administration," he explained. He lost weight and became a dashing young man. Three years later he moved to Albany, where he found a job with a state councilman. He was moving up in the world, fulfilling his dream.

LOW SELF-ESTEEM

◇ Proud to Be Who She Is

"It's time to do soul retrieval to find the source of that block," I suggested to Johanna, a successful writer in her midthirties. "Yes, I'd like to do it," she said. "I want to find out what stopped me from being proud of who I am." I asked her to lie down, and I sat by her side, lightly touching her hand with my knee, and started drumming.

I called my power animal, and we flew high into the blue sky. We hovered over a forest with a few houses on the edge of it. Looking down, I noticed a group of children playing on the left side of my vision field. I came closer and saw a blond short girl dressed in a nice light "girly" dress, standing in anguish and disbelieve. An older, tall blond boy was telling her something very nasty. I could not tell what he was saying. Immediately, he and another smaller boy ran away to the right of her and disappeared into the woods. By her side I noticed another younger girl. "Maybe her sister?" I thought.

I took a look at the surroundings. Somehow, I knew it was their secret hiding place under a large tree; its long roundabout green branches made it look like a mysterious cavern. I looked at the girl again. She was frozen in shock, as if she realized that she could not be liked. A thought came to my mind. "Maybe he told her she couldn't be a boy because she doesn't have a penis like him and the other younger boy." I felt her deep confusion, sadness, and disappointment.

I went looking for her lost soul part. My eyes were drawn to the top of the tree where I discovered two young chicks in a small nest huddling together. Their open mouths were loudly calling their mother to be fed. I recognized one of the chicks as Johanna. I asked her permission to bring her back with me, so she could reunite with her older self. To my surprise she agreed easily. I stopped drumming, raised my hands, and held her in the palms of my hands and then proceeded to blow her into Johanna's heart and then her crown.

"Wow, I remember this event very well, although I haven't thought of it since I was five or six years old." "That is usually what happens in a soul loss, to avoid the trauma pain," I explained her. "We used to play in that secret place in that small forest near my house. I even remember the names of the two brothers. I remember the painful sad feeling I had then when he was verbally abusing me. I did not understand his cruelty." Johanna was obviously moved. She took a big breath and continued. "What you have seen makes sense to me. I always felt different from the other boys or girls. I was like a stranger, as if I could not be normal like all the others. Later in life, in college, I discovered that I am attracted to women. It was so difficult and confusing. I am okay with that now. It makes sense that in some situations I am afraid that people will ridicule me, and I feel like hiding. My girlfriend now is very supportive of me."

◇ Cinderella: Soul Retrieval

"Yes, I am from Istanbul. I heard about you from my friend who had a session with you there. I am very nervous and anxious and can't sleep because I have to go back home to meet my family and apply for a job with a very important person in my field," said Maral, a young woman. "Why are you so anxious?" I asked her. "They criticize me all the time, especially my older sister. She makes me feel like I am a stupid outcast." "What are you doing here?" I asked her. "I am an architect. I worked in Istanbul for many years and now here, but my visa is up," she said. "Surely you can't be stupid to be doing this work," I said with a laugh. "I don't think I am, but my family treats me like I am nothing." She was upset. "Let's do a candle and palm reading so we can see what's going on." She agreed. After the readings I felt that we needed to do soul retrieval, and she agreed to try.

I sat by her side as she lay down and I started drumming. Closing my eyes, I called my power animal for help, and after our short exchange, he took me to see a skinny girl about seven or eight years old standing in front of an old stone house covered by deteriorating plaster. She stood there in her simple white dress by a tree, frozen and unable to move. The girl watched her father and sister walking toward a black car that was waiting in the driveway. They left without acknowledging her. "This must be what Cinderella felt as she saw her stepmother and her stepsisters going to the king's ball," I thought to myself. As the car left, the little girl dug a large hole in the earth in front of her, wanting to bury herself and disappear from this life. I felt so sad for her.

I took a look into the little crater. There was a small green plant growing, reaching up to the sun. Maybe it is a sign that her life is about to change for the better, I thought to myself. Immediately a little green and brown frog leaped closer and stood at the edge of the hole. "Who are you?" I asked her. "I am the soul part Maral lost," the frog said. "She needs to feel loved again. If you want you may carry me to her, but first you need to show me love and give me a kiss." I held her in my hands, brought her to my lips and kissed the rough skin of the back of her shoulders and head. To my true surprise the frog shape shifted into a beautiful tiny princess with a white dress and a red cap. It was a beautiful sight. "Would you be ready now to join Maral in her heart?" I asked her. "Yes, I am ready," the little princes said, smiling broadly. Just before I lay down my drum, a very brilliant shooting star with a long tail illuminated the sky, as if it wanted to let me know that her ancestors were watching and that she was protected, which surprised me. I bent down above my client and blew the little princess into her heart three times, and then I helped her sit up and blew it three times into the crown of her head. We sat facing each other.

"I must tell you that I had a strange vision almost like a children's fairytale. I don't know if it will make any sense to you," I confessed. She looked at me with her big dark eyes in anticipation. I watched her face twisted in pain with tears in her eyes as I went on to describe my vision.

"It's true. I remember that time, very well," Maral said, with deep pain in her voice and her black eyes. "I was six then," she corrected me.

"I remember the white dress. It was my favorite, and I used to wear a red headband in my hair. That day I wanted to just disappear. I remember looking at the earth and wanting to bury myself so no one would know I existed." She took a big breath and wiped her tears. "Yes, we lived in that house like you described. At the entrance stood one old tree. We had a black car, like you saw. My father always preferred my sister to me. He used to leave me by myself many times. I don't think he ever loved me." We sat in quietness. "I think we need to do the cleansing ceremony and I would like you to bring up that six-year-old girl and ask her what she needs you to do to be integrated into your life."

The next day she wrote: "Dear Itzhak, Thank you very much for the healing yesterday. I am very well. I slept for almost fifteen hours after the healing. I woke up and wrote my CV again more courageously and wrote to some potential business partners I had avoided for a long time. The very bright light you had seen at the end of the session can be my ancestor and spirit teacher I mentioned you about. Rumi is my ancestor (from my grandfather's family), and I always ask for his help in my shamanic journeys. I did not mention his name, but you had seen this very bright light, and in my opinion, it can be Rumi. Is it possible?"

A few weeks later I received another e-mail. "Hello Itzhak, Just to let you know I am feeling very well after the soul retrieval. I believe I changed a lot. My job interviews are going very well with a lot of synchronicity. And my sister is very nice to me! See you soon in New York."

LIFE CONFUSION

◇ Message from Her Ancestor

"I am an energy healer, a reiki master, but I don't feel I am doing the work I came here to do. I know there is something else for me," my client told me as we sat facing each other. She was tall and pale, with very short blond hair and dark eyes. "I want more clarity on my direction," she said.

What came next was amazing. A strange vision that changed her life and that afterward would take her on a trip with me to the Brazilian

Amazon to be initiated into the power of a Shaore, a Kanamari tribal shaman.

I performed a cleansing ceremony. As it progressed, with my open eyes I saw an image of a dark, old owl face hovering just above her head. Mesmerized by the image I looked closely and discovered it was not an owl. It was actually a wrinkled old woman, burned dark by the sun. She had big piercing black eyes and wore a black scarf around her head.

"Who are you?" I asked her telepathically. "I am your client's great-great-great-grandmother." "Where are you from?" I asked her. "I am from Sicily, south of Italy." "Why are you here?" I asked. "I need to teach her to be a witch, a medicine woman, like me, so she could continue my work." I was dumbfounded. How could it be? My client looked Swedish. I decided to ask her.

I stopped the ceremony. "Marie, are you not a natural blond? Did your family come from Sicily?" I asked her. Surprised and confused, she immediately answered, "Oh no, I color my hair. It is naturally black. Why do you ask?" I shared with her that her ancestor is here, and the message she wanted me to tell her. "Oh, that is so strange. Yes, my family emigrated from Sicily. I heard some stories that some women in my family line used to do magic and healing," she said. We both took a deep breath and relaxed again, and then I went on with the ceremony.

Without waiting the old woman ancestor was back. This time she instructed me in a sacred women fire ceremony she used to officiate. "Tell this to Marie," she insisted. "This is a late night ceremony, at midnight is best, when all the men are in their beds sleeping. Put eight large square stones around the bonfire, in each direction and in between them. Each woman stands by her stone; she becomes the guardian of her direction." I saw them, like in a movie, chanting rhythmically, and then they began to move around the fire, holding small tambourines in one hand and sticks in the other. When the time was right, the women stood in line and walked barefoot over the hot coals and finally extinguished the fire with their bare feet. "Tell her we do this ceremony to foster women's resilience and personal power. It brings us to connect intimately with the fire, which is the symbol of the female sexuality," she instructed me. And then she disappeared, vanished back into her time. It was such a privilege to be used as an instrument to bring messages and connection between generations of healers. I shared this message with Marie.

My client followed up on her ancestor's message. She became a shaman practitioner and in her work she empowers other women in groups and individually.

◇ Holy Man

"I am fighting unwanted forces, my life is unraveling under me, and I am so stressful. My financial situation is bad, my business is falling apart, and my partner and I are separating. It seems I need your help." So Jonathan wrote me in his e-mail.

"Faith, faith, faith, the candle indicates that you lost the belief in yourself and trust in the universe. You need to get back to yourself, to peruse what is really important in life, without fear; you must tap back into your spiritual practices and use them," I told the handsome, desperate, middle-aged man sitting across from me. "It's true; I feel lost right now, even though I try to keep positive and meditate," he said in agony. "Now, let's remove this dark cloud of negative energy from you," I suggested. "Please take off your clothes, stand in the center of the room, and face me. Close your eyes and take a deep breath. Release everything you are holding onto into the stones in your hands. I will let you know when to open your eyes," I instructed him.

I took my place a few steps away from him, raised the bottle of trago, and called the mountain spirits to help us in the ceremony. I scanned his body energy carefully and slowly closed my eyes before blowing the sugarcane rum over him. Instantaneously, an image appeared above his third eye of an orange-pink flower, a lotus. In the center of that lotus, I noticed a blue god smiling at me. His body and hands seemed to be moving in a ritualistic dance. "It must be a Hindu god," I thought. "But what is he doing here above my client's head?" I wondered.

I opened my eyes and asked my client if he is a follower or a believer of an Indian blue god. He opened his eyes in surprise. "Oh, yes. I lived with my guru in his ashram in India for a few years, and we worshipped Krishna, who is the blue god," he said. I felt a bit embarrassed for not recognizing Krishna. "Why do you ask?" He was curious. "Well, he is here above your head, in the center of a lotus flower," I answered. We both laughed. "Okay, let's start again," I told him.

I closed my eyes, ready to blow the trago again. To my astonishment Krishna started to communicate with me: "Please tell your client that his life's mission is to bring enlightenment to people everywhere."

Again, I opened my eyes and presented that message to my client. "Yes, as you may know Krishna is the god of enlightenment," Jonathan confirmed. "I am not surprised by this message, " he said laughing. "Okay. Let's start again," I said for the third time.

I closed my eyes—ready to blow the trago and start the ceremony— and again another image came in, except that this time I saw above the beautiful orange lotus, where Krishna was still sitting, a white bright spirit. It descended from above, like a white transparent sheet of light. It hugged my client and enveloped him in its soft touch. I was mesmerized by the spirit and looked carefully at it. It had a mane of white long hair, and it was weaving lightly in the wind from side to side. I could not tell if it was a male or a female or both. "That is really strange; who could that be?" I asked myself, not wanting to be embarrassed again.

I opened my eyes for the fourth time and described to Jonathan what I just witnessed, "Oh, that is Malki Tzedek, the biblical angel I'm working with now. How amazing." "You must be very lucky to have all these powerful spiritual teachers around to help you. Use them, connect with them, trust them; I think they want you to start a whole new chapter now." I suggested to him after the cleansing ceremony was over. "You are so right. I got so distracted and far away from them." He promised to renew his practice.

◇ Her Healing in Her Own Words

Curious to understand why my clients came to see me in the first place, how they found the experience of shamanic healing, and if the experience changed their lives, I asked them if they could share their healing journeys with me. One of my clients, Magdalena, wonderfully described the intimate process she went through.

"When I first came to see you I felt extremely lost in my life. I stayed in New York for about one year, instead of the originally planned three-month stay, because I fell in love with somebody. After this relationship ended I went back to my home country but had no further plans for my life. I could actually have gotten back into my old life where I had a great job, but some irrational voice told me to go back to the United States. So I left my country without much money, without having a visa, and without knowing exactly what I would do there. Once I was back in New York, I completely lost my footing. Everything turned into a nightmare in my exterior and interior life. I felt like I was floating and lost in space, and I got depressed and anxious. I had to admit to myself that I needed help to become oriented and to reconnect with myself."

"Why have you chosen shamanic healing over other methods?" I asked her.

"I never believed in school medicine and always tried to avoid any prescriptions that were given to me. Since I was trained as a dancer I knew that the body and the mind are connected. I realized that if something isn't working well, you couldn't talk it away or make it to go away by taking a pill. A human is a whole complex being, and it never made sense to me to focus on just the one part that isn't functioning. One example is my first—and last—visit at a psychologist's office. Somebody recommended that I go there since I was dragging a lot of pain from my childhood with me. The woman made me talk about everything that went wrong in my childhood, and after an hour her alarm reminded her that my time was over. She let me go with an immense overwhelming feeling of despair and set up an appointment for next week. The whole meeting felt really wrong to me, and I realized that talking is not what I need. I felt like there is a space surrounding me that makes my emotional well-being unreachable through only talking. Talking felt as if I were drinking milk to cure diarrhea; forgive me but that is the only metaphor that came to my mind. It felt like it made the problem increase instead of decrease. I believe in shamanic healing because I can feel and see things shifting within myself. I can't really explain in words exactly what is happening with me, but I trust in this method of healing and also think we don't need to be able to explain everything with words. My regular physician is also an alternative healer. She lived with indigenous tribes in the south of Mexico and has seen and learned a lot there. I'm so happy I got to meet her because through her I got introduced to shamanism. She is not practicing shamanic healing, but she has her own garden where she grows healing plants, and she makes her own plant tinctures for her patients. She is a trained physician but includes a lot of shamanic techniques into her practice. For example, she always tries to figure out where your illness is coming from. She asks good questions, which make you think about possible relations to your illness. She only prescribes Western medication if something is very serious and you need immediate relief or treatment. What I love about her is that she takes time for you. I think the way that we treat time in Western society is also a huge factor related to illness or problems."

"Can you describe your first session experience with me and those that followed?" I asked her.

"My first session was very interesting. The first thing you did was a candle reading. I was blown away by how much you told me about myself without previously having chatted with me! Then you did a cleansing session with me. I had had a cleansing session once before with the Mexican shamans of the International Council of Thirteen Indigenous Grandmothers, but that was very different. Later on I also had some journeys and soul retrievals in your sessions. I was surprised that the cleansing session was kind of a performance. I had to laugh to myself, and I remember thinking, 'Here I am, feeling completely lost in New York, and now I somehow managed to land in some shaman's office who is spitting alcohol all over me.' Anyway, I managed to relax and just let things happen. My reaction after the first session was awful. For one week, I stayed in my bedroom. I couldn't stop crying, my legs were aching, and I had a terrible flu. I really went through one of the worst times of my life! I remember calling you and telling you that I can't stop crying and that I'm afraid of what is happening. You said that

I have a lot of pain stored in my body, and it needs to be released and that I shouldn't worry and just let it happen. After I hung up I didn't feel much better or safer with this answer, but what else could I do? I had no close friends in the city, and for some reason I didn't want to contact anybody back home and tell them what was happening. So I managed to let things happen, and eventually I started feeling better. I had two more sessions shortly after the first one and was slowly feeling stronger again; although I remember it took a lot of courage to go back and have more sessions after my strong reaction to the first one."

"What was the one important experience or learning you had that was relevant to your life?" I asked her.

"Again, it was proven to me that there is something else surrounding our bodies that can't be removed by talking or taking pills. I think, in general, I became more and more aware of the interconnectedness of things—the body, the soul, energies, the people, the whole world, just simply everything. Before this experience, I saw myself as a single puzzle piece that didn't fit into the puzzle. This experience also brought many other consequences. Because I'm feeling more connected, I'm starting to be very concerned about our environment and about what is happening in the world. I used to feel much more detached about all that. I guess that is a good thing, but I have to learn how to deal with this concern."

"What were the short- and long-term results?"

"Well, I'd say this is a short- and long-term result. Shortly after this whole process with you, I met my husband, with whom I'm still happily married today. I don't think that could have ever happened with all the pain that I had been dragging with me from my childhood. My previous relationships always fell apart and added even more to my pain. It was a pattern in my life that I never was able to break through. I felt desperate for many years not being able to manage and change this. I also started a retail business, something I could not have imagined doing before, and it is still going well. I'm learning to be tough."

"In what way did this experience change you and the people around you?" was my next question.

"I feel that it shifted my perspective big time. Before this experience

I was kind of more on a treadmill of constantly wondering how to do something right. I felt from early on that people in my surroundings always wanted me to do things the right way. I always wanted to be accepted, so I would bend myself and try to do things the 'right way' according to what I thought was expected of me. It was really frustrating because I felt I was never able to do things right. I guess the frustration also had to do with my need for recognition and appreciation. After seeing you I started to accept myself more for how I am. I don't feel wrong so often anymore. I don't try to censor myself all the time anymore. I would say the experience with you changed my relationship with my inner self and that affects my relationships with the people around me."

ANXIETY

◆ Facing Her Trauma

"I wanted to see you because in two weeks I am going to visit my family in Italy. Lately I feel so angry. I lash out at my husband and blame him for everything. I hate this about myself. I know it's not his fault; he is a really good man. I know he loves me. I am frightened because I am also impatient with my two-year-old daughter. I don't like to see myself doing this, but I can't help it. I want to know what's going on with me. Why is this happening to me?" asked Maura when we met again, a few months after our first session. Maura, a tall woman with beautiful brown curly hair, always has a big smile on her face but today she was distraught.

"Tell me, why are you going to Italy?" I asked her. "I need to visit my parents. They are very upset. They just lost their restaurant. They have no money and have huge debts. I feel like I need to work harder to bring money with me to help them, as they have helped me in the past," she said with fear in her voice. "Did they tell you that?" I asked. "No, my sister told me. They did not want to worry me. They always want to protect me from bad news," she replied and fiddled with her fingers.

"Can you remember another time in your childhood that something like that happened?" I asked her. "No, no, I can't remember anything like that," she said after a minute. I looked at her sad brown eyes and scanned her energy field above her head. A vision with a clear message came. "What happened to you when you were seven or eight years old? I can see that you had a frightening trauma around that age. Can you recall that memory?" I carefully asked her, trying to confirm the message I received.

She lowered her head and looked down at the floor. I could see she was straining to remember. We sat a few minutes quietly. All of a sudden she raised her head and exclaimed. "Wow, yes, I remember. You are right. When I was that age, my parents had a big financial crisis. They never told me directly anything. I guess they tried to protect me, just like today. But I sensed that something horrible had happened. I listen to their hushed phone conversations with the people whom they owed money to. I was scared and terrified; I did not know what to do. I could not ask them either. I can't believe I remember it now. It is exactly like what is happening now," she said. "Except that you are now a grown-up at thirty-two, and you have your own family," I reminded her. A big smile spread on her face. "Let's do a short exercise," I suggested. "Close your eyes. Can you see that little girl?" "Yes." "Where is she?"

"She is standing on a staircase, holding the metal rails with her hands, listening from above. I see my parents quarreling. I think it is about money."

"What are you wearing?" "A red jumpsuit." She smiled at the image.

"Do you like that little girl?" Her face squirmed with repulsion. "No, she is very sad and scared; I don't like it," she replied.

"Can you see her eyes? What do you see?" "Innocence. Powerlessness. Despair."

"Can you tell her that you, at your age, can take care of her now?" I continued.

"I did, but she doesn't believe me." Her face was disappointed.

"Can you ask her if she would like to be hugged?"

"She said that she doesn't want it. She doesn't trust me." Tears started rolling down her face.

"Ask her if there is anything that she needs from her parents."

"She says that she wants unconditional love and safety."

"Can you offer this to her now?"

"Yes, I did."

"Is she smiling now?"

"Yes."

"Can you ask her if she would like to be hugged now?"

"Yes, she agrees."

"How does it feel in your body?"

"Wonderful and warm."

"Where do you feel it in your body?"

"Here", and she put her hand on her heart and belly.

"Good. Can you now sing her your favorite lullaby?"

"Okay, I'll try." I watched her as she was singing. She rocked the little girl from side to side. A sweet smile appeared on her face; she was transformed into a soft motherly Madonna.

"Would you ask her if she wants to join you in your heart?"

"She is already there."

"Wonderful. Can you promise her that you will always be there for her anytime she needs you?"

"Yes, I did."

"Can you give her permission to let you know when she feels unloved, frightened, and unsafe? Can you promise her you will check on her from time to time to make sure she is okay?"

"Yes."

"Would you like to say good-bye for now until you meet again?"

"I did." And she smiled.

"You can open your eyes."

Maura sat with a big wide smile on her face, wiping the tears from her cheeks. "It was so simple. I could not believe that that incident had so much impact on my life. Thank you."

"Now we need to do one more thing. I would like you to do a shamanic journey with your power animal to meet your parents' spirits. Ask them what is it that they want from you when you come to visit them," I suggested. "Okay, that sounds good." And so we did. She lay on the blanket, and I drummed for her.

"My power animal took me to the upper world where I met them. They were truly happy to see me. I asked them the question. To my surprise they did not ask for money; they said they want me and my daughter to bring happiness and joy, nothing more."

Maura left our session and went back to her waiting husband and daughter full of optimism, relief, and joy. "I am so happy I came to see you before I left," she exclaimed as we said good-bye.

◈ Taking Responsibility

With her right hand Lena opened the door as quickly as she could. Then she turned around and faced me. "So you say it was all my fault," she exclaimed and burst out laughing sarcastically as she grabbed her bag and headed out the door. I could see a small tear at the corner of her eye. It had been an intense session. "Not your fault, more like your responsibility," I said before bidding her good-bye. Maybe I was too rough on her. She will not come back again, I thought to myself. Oh well, sometimes you just have to tell the truth.

As I took a big breath, another massage therapist case from a few years back came rushing to my mind. One Sunday morning, Rachel, an Upper West Side, middle-aged, elegant woman, refused my request to take some of her clothes off for the cleansing ceremony. I was surprised. I turned around toward my altar to grab the bottle of rum to start the ceremony and sarcastically muttered under my breath, "Well, massage therapist . . ." "What did you say?" she screamed. "I said I was surprised that a massage therapist refuses to take off her clothes," I answered calmly looking in her eyes. She stood a few feet away from me, put her hands on her hips, and cursed me out with full vigor, stomping her feet on the floor. I was shocked. A tsunami of emotions flew through me. But I did not respond, letting her vent. When she quieted down, I asked her calmly if she wanted to continue with our ceremony. She reluctantly agreed and I went on, truthfully a bit shaken.

When she sat down after the ceremony, her face and eyes were glowing. "Thank you! she said. I was surprised. "I was always afraid to stand my ground in front of my father and my husband. Thank you for allowing me the space to do it. I feel such relief." We became fast friends and she returned for more sessions and even sent her husband and son to see me as well.

My current client, Lena, a tall and beautiful woman in her late thirties, was also a massage therapist, working for a wellness center in one of the largest corporations in the city. "Everyone hates me. They all talk about me behind my back. They spread rumors that make my regular clients leave me," were some of her common complaints, which we had been working on for a few months now. It was always somebody else's faults. Never hers. She refused to take any blame. That day something had changed. She was able to hear this from her power animal during a shamanic journey in the spirit world. She asked questions and she got an answer she did not expect.

Two weeks passed after she stormed out of my office and she came back to her next session. I was surprised. "I came to thank you. I don't think I am going to come back for some time now, but I needed you to know that things at my work have shifted." This time there was no sarcasm in her voice. "Tell me," I encouraged her. "I don't know, but they are all much nicer to me; my old clients came back too." "Do you think it has to do with you?" I asked her. "Yes, yes, it was entirely my fault," she laughed.

I suggested we would do a journey to meet her mother's soul so she could heal that painful relationship. She agreed. And we sealed it with another cleansing ceremony before she went away.

◇ Cutting the Cords

I received the following e-mail from Lorna: "I am going through a very difficult custody case and could really use some help with the negative energy surrounding me. I would be interested in a session with you." We set up a time and a well-dressed businesswoman showed up; from the look of her you would think everything in her life was perfect. But it turns out that wasn't the case. My candle reading indicated fear, fear, and more fear. Because of her need to be liked she always chose partners who took advantage of her and manipulated her to take care of them without contributing to the partnership themselves.

"I was afraid to let them go; I was afraid they would be violent with me and I needed company," she said when she realized her pattern after we did soul retrieval. She healed the part of herself that needed a woman's approval and felt the deep fear of emotional abandonment by her mother. In the few sessions we had, we used many of shamanic tools, such as soul retrieval, shamanic journeys with the help of spirit guides, La Limpia ceremonies, guided journeys, and cord cutting, which was very hard for her to do. At the end she got what she wanted: full custody of her daughter and the legal release of her previous partner.

She was a free woman at last. Here is the e-mail I received from her after all of this:

Hi, Itzhak,
I wanted to let you know what happened to me one week post severing of my ex's tie to me [cord-cutting ceremony]. . . . I went to court, and out of the blue, the judge severed my ex's rights! She didn't physically appear, and so I was awarded sole custody with all of her visitation rights suspended and a two-year full stay-away order of protection for my daughter! Honestly, I have been in court for four years over this. My attorney is in shock and said that this never happens in court. Thank you for all that you have done for me.

And then she later sent a thank you note: "I don't know why I came to see you in the first place. Maybe I was desperate. I tried lawyers, counselors, and the 'normal' ways. But nothing happened. After each of our sessions something strange happened. After the first one I found pennies everywhere even in places I could not imagine. After the second session I found dimes everywhere, and after the third I found feathers everywhere. Isn't it strange? I think there is magic in what you do. Or maybe my awareness became wider and larger? Yes, I feel so."

OTHER MENTAL AND EMOTIONAL CONDITIONS

◈ *Panic Attacks: Recovering the Warrior Soul*

My healer friend John, a great multitalented healer, called me one day. "I can't help this client of mine anymore. I've seen her every week for a few years now, but she is really stuck. Maybe you can do something for her using your shamanic techniques." He sounded obviously frustrated. He knew my work as he himself had experienced it a few times. "I can't promise anything, but I'll try my best. It's in spirit hands," I told him, wondering why he gave up on her. That is how Elisabeth came into my life some twelve years ago.

Elisabeth had been suffering from panic attacks and insomnia, among many other ills. It took three years of sessions, but eventually this retired high school teacher and single mother completely changed her life, though she continues to come for monthly "maintenance sessions" as we call them. She no longer suffers from weekly debilitating late-night panic attacks. No longer has difficulty falling asleep. And no longer lashes out at people around her. "Many years as a public school teacher can do that," she once said sarcastically. Even her eyebrows have started to grow back—another one of her symptoms.

Elisabeth swore off using medication or visiting regular doctors. She had a strong belief in alternative and natural medicine and her ability to heal herself. I did not do it alone: she created a team of alternative healers who supported her on her healing journey. To keep herself busy she started taking painting and voice lessons and cultivated a small group of female friends. These friendships have helped to make up for the loss of her only sister. In our sessions she shared how her family had left her alone and how difficult it was to find a life partner.

She now regularly goes to a gym to keep herself in shape and is very proud of it. "I don't like to be around people my age. They all look so old and are always talking about sickness and medicines," she said. She has become a successful painter and now shows and sells her work in galleries and museums around the world. She even overcame her fear of computers and built her own website. She frequently travels, although she is still afraid of flying, and has a full social calendar. It took much work for Elisabeth to overcome her many fears and emotional difficulties.

Diagnostic Reading

On my first session with Elisabeth, I asked this medium-height, red-headed, full-sized woman to rub a white candle all over her body to let it absorb her energy. I lit it and took a look at the flame. The large blue area had a dark cloud and a large black mass revealing a strong-willed and powerful woman, but also a woman who possessed deep fears and who had endured a trauma and perhaps a soul loss, perhaps at three or four years of age. It appeared to be sexual abuse and was currently manifesting as digestive problems. Looking higher on the wick I could see that her voice and throat were blocked and that she might have a thyroid problem. "Is that true?" I asked her. "I don't remember my early childhood, only vaguely. I have a suspicion that something bad happened," she said. "I take natural supplements for my thyroid, and it helps a little, and yes, I always have had digestive problems, and I'm always bloated." She sighed.

Relieved, I went on with my reading. "I can see one blond-haired sister. You have an especially close relationship with her." She started to weep. "It's true. She died two years ago, and I feel so lonely without her." We sat quietly as she sobbed. I concentrated on the flame again. "A skinny red-headed man, a negative spirit, is hanging around you. This may be your father. Not a very communicative guy," I said, and she nodded her head in agreement. "Your apartment is stuffy and has no plants or flowers. You must change that," I told her. "I've tried, believe me. But the plants die from too much heat and the lack of light. I'll try again," she said. "You are also out of balance with regard to your creativity. You think too much. Physically you have strong legs," I finished. "Okay. Can I see the palms of your hands now?"

As I glanced over her hands, it was obvious she was a passionate, stubborn doer and a leader who needs complete independence. "You dislike people who tell you what to do and can't stand needy people.

Is that right?" I asked her. "I just can't stand stupid people," she sighed. "You are very intuitive with a strong need and ability for self-expression. Do you express yourself?" I asked her. "Just a little. I paint a little and take voice lessons, but it goes nowhere."

She took a big breath, looked down, and softly said, "I believe I was sexually abused or inappropriately touched as a young girl but can't remember it. Yes, I want to be in a relationship with a man, but I can't trust them. The man who got me pregnant left." She lifted her eyes and looked in mine. "My sister and I were extremely close, and I miss her so much. There were a lot of losses in a very short time in my life. I lost my mom, aunt, and most importantly my sister to cancer. And now my son is moving out, leaving too."

And then she added "Since I am afraid of flying, I was not able to get to my sister's funeral. I blame my brother-in-law for not waiting for me to come by train from New York to Los Angeles. How could he do this to me? He did it on purpose." She was in grief for not being able to say a proper good-bye to her only sister and had become obsessed in her hatred of her brother-in-law.

Sister Is Back

At one of our next sessions as I performed La Limpia, the energy-cleansing ceremony, her younger sister's spirit showed up as a hologram, above and to the left of her. Wearing an all-white dress she was calmly swinging under a large tree in the backyard of her house. As she swung up and down, her long blond curly hair floated in the air; she had a beautiful and peaceful smile on her young face. "Let Elisabeth know that I am in peace," she said. And then a new image appeared in which I saw my client playing with her sister, who idolized her to no end.

"It's so good to know she is around me," my client cried with great relief.

Before she left I prescribed traditional dietary restrictions for her and asked her to do candle meditations, reorganize her crowded apartment, and bring new plants and flowers home. I also suggested she take sea-salt baths, and whenever she felt that familiar feeling of anxiety returning, she should hold a stone in each hand and breathe. Elisabeth promised she would follow my instructions, and she did. I admire her for her commitment to her healing.

Burial Ceremony

After a few more sessions, Elisabeth realized that her life was controlled by anger, despair, and feelings of powerlessness. I suggested we would do a special ceremony of anger release. "OK, if you think it will help." She sounded resigned. "Write a letter to your sister," I said. "To my sister? She's already dead. Why should I write to her?" she asked. "Tell her all the things you were not able to tell her before she passed on. Everything. Don't worry about grammar or spelling. Do it in your own handwriting, and please do not go back and re-read it and make corrections. At the same time please write a second letter." "To whom?" she asked. "To your brother-in-law."

Elisabeth looked at me surprised and quite irritated. "I hate him," she murmured. "Yes, I know. That is why you need to do it," I said.

Two weeks later, in a small nearby park surrounded by tall apartments buildings, she performed the burial ceremony. Quietly hidden among a thick group of small trees, avoiding the sharp park-keeper eyes, chanting, and making a special prayer and offerings, she dug a hole in the soft soil of Mother Earth, pulled out two fat white envelopes, and slowly burned each handwritten page. As we watched them dissolve into ashes, she prayed for the release of the anger, disillusions, hopes, and attachment she was holding against her family. Then quietly with her two hands she covered the ashes with fresh soil.

The following session Elisabeth came in looking a whole lot different. That angry, impatient, and disappointed part of her was no longer there. She looked calm and at peace. "I don't understand it, but I'm no longer angry with him or with my sister. I think I disconnected from them somehow. I am just really, deeply sad," she said quietly. We sat on either side of my altar for a long while in total quietness, allowing her to be with her sorrow and experience her grieving. There were no tears. There was nothing to say or do. She fully surrendered.

"Would you like me to teach you how to do a shamanic journey so you can communicate with your sister?" I asked her at the next session. "I can't do it," she protested, claiming that although she regularly attends the monthly New York Shamanic Circle she has never been successful in seeing visions. "Spirit speaks to us in many ways. Everyone sees differently," I told her. "Some see images, some feel, some experience body sensations, some hear voices, and some just have explicit knowing," I continued. "Let's try it." We did, and she successfully acquired a power animal and is using it whenever she needs it.

Soul Retrieval

"I think you are now ready to find out the source of your trauma," I told her at one session. She looked surprised. I explained what a soul retrieval ceremony is and how we were going to do it. "Would you like to try to do it?" "Okay, I trust you."

She lay on the blanket and covered her eyes as I sat by her side, lightly touching her arm. I started drumming rapidly calling my spirit guide for help on this task. I was immediately taken to a small dusty town. There, on the stairs in front of a small apartment building, were sitting two young girls, maybe two and four years old, dressed in travel clothes, waiting. Big suitcases surrounded them. There was some commotion around them.

Then my vision took me to long and wide sand dunes. "Where is this? Am I making this up? Where are they going?" I asked and doubted myself. A new vision appeared. I found the four-year-old girl on a ship. She was in a completely dark room, all by herself and full of fear, as the boat was violently rocking from side to side, tossing her like a leaf in a storm. Terrified, she was screaming for help, but no one was able to hear her. My body clasped with emotional pain.

I then asked my spirit guide to help me find her lost soul part, which she let go of to survive that horrific trauma. My power animal took me to a corner of the ceiling above her bed. There, stuck in the corner I met a little frightened doll. I introduced myself first and tried to convince her to reunite with big Elisabeth, but she refused. "I don't want to. It's not safe," she said. I persuaded her that my client is now old enough to take care of her and told her of her great accomplishments and that she can be proud of her.

She was still suspicious, but finally agreed to come back. I stopped drumming and held her in the palms of my hands. I bent over Elisabeth and blew it right into her heart. Then I helped her to sit up and blew it into the crown of her head. We sat quietly for a few minutes.

"What did you see?" she asked as we sat down facing each other. She listened carefully as I told her my vision. Her response surprised me, as it happens many times that I myself was incredibly skeptical of my own visions and messages from spirit.

"It was true. I do not remember it clearly, but my parents told me this story too. We were migrating from Tel Aviv to South America where we had some relatives, first by train to the port of Alexandria in Egypt. The long train ride was through the Sinai Desert. And then we boarded a ship. One night my parents, perhaps thinking I was asleep, left me alone and went out to the deck, maybe to go dancing. All of a sudden a huge storm began. I was tossed from side to side. It was completely dark and nobody heard my cries or came to help me. Since then I could not trust the world or them and never felt safe again, always waiting for the worst to happen."

She stopped. "Do you think that this is the reason for my panic attacks?" she asked. Mulling it over in her mind, she continued, "Maybe this is why I get frozen at night?"

"I think we should do a journey to welcome her back," I suggested. I suggested that Elisabeth find a chorus to sing with so that she could learn to release her fear of expressing herself and to give her a chance to be around a community of people. I also recommended that since she has leadership qualities she could gather her artist friends and organize art shows and maybe painting trips.

She joined a church and began singing in the church's chorus, where she became the most dominant voice there. She started using her leadership qualities by organizing a few group exhibitions and painting trips with her friends. She's even considering flying. She sure has gained control over her life.

Artist's Statement

"Elisabeth, why are painting the way you do?" I asked her on one of our sessions. She looked surprised. "I don't know. I just like strong colors with large movements," she hesitantly replied.

"Think about it. What is your artist statement? What do you want a visitor to your website to know about you or what do you want to say to gallery owners you are pitching your work to?" I continued to press on her. "I never thought about it. Is it important?" she asked.

"Your paintings are an expression of your inner world. They communicate the true essence of your soul. Can you put that into simple words?" I asked her. "When you paint, are you trying to cover up your anxiety and fear or are you communicating your excitement and love of life? Where does the inspiration to paint them come from?" She looked puzzled.

"Here is your homework. Write down your artist statement in two paragraphs. And bring it to our next session," I told her. And so she did. "I never thought that being born in Israel and moving to South America and then to California and Arizona had so much influence on my color pallet," she said on our next session. She read from her artist statement: "Creating my art allows me to forget all of my life's torments. I am infusing my inner world with joyous bright colors and strong motions, energy that activates the universe and all of life."

◇ Schizophrenia: Opening and Closing the Gate

The phone rang in my office. On the other end was a worried mother. "I don't know exactly what you do, but you were highly recommended by a friend who saw you before. Can you also help my daughter? She has schizophrenia. Can I come with her and stay at the session? She can't take the train from Long Island by herself," the anxious mother said. "Sure," I assured her, "and you can stay throughout the session if she agrees." We set up the time and I hung up.

An upsetting memory of another schizophrenic client crossed my mind. It was of an older woman, an author and college professor. In one of our sessions she shot up from her chair, claiming spirit told her to show me a particular dance. There was no way to convince her to sit or to calm her down. Frenzied, she removed some of her clothes and wildly galloped and hopped in big round movements across the room, circling the air with multicolored silk scarfs she had pulled from her bag, as if she were the legendary modern dancer Isadora Duncan. All the while she accompanied herself with uninhibited singing. So of course I was a bit concerned for what I would encounter with this next client.

"I hear voices all the time," Jennifer said, hugging her elbows tightly, her eyes gazing down, as we sat down by my altar. "They always tell me what to do and what to think, many time with opposing instructions. If I protest, they laugh and ridicule me. It is so confusing. This is why I can't decide where to go and what to do." I saw the deep desperation in the eyes of this beautiful light-haired young woman. She raised her eyes and looked at me. "Do you think you can you help me?" she asked quietly.

"When did you first start hearing the voices?" I asked her. She thought for a minute. "It started a few years ago, before college. First there were short messages. I thought I was making it up, maybe because of the school pressure, and then it got worse, almost nonstop. Now I sit in my house and don't go out. I'm so confused and so tired." She continued to hug herself tightly.

"In indigenous societies, people who have your condition are not stigmatized as mentally sick, as they are in our culture," I explained. "Instead they are revered as they have a special power to make a direct connection to spirits, and many times it is a sign that they can become shamans or healers to their community. No one knows why spirits choose those special people." I watched the surprise spread across her face. "Sometimes, spirits do overtake and possess a person's body, but as far as I can see you do not have that," I told her.

She was trying to understand what I just said. "So, they are not sick?" she asked. "No, they just have easy access to what we call the spirit world or ancestors," I assured her. "Sometime it is can also be manifested in a physical form, like in what we call epileptic seizures. In the Mongolian and Tibetan traditions, epilepsy is a symptom of a person who is called by spirit to become a shaman or a seer. In many cases when the person fully surrenders to the calling and embraces it, the physical manifestations cease, and the person is healed," I added.

I suggested that we first do a candle reading. "In the candle flame I can see you have a great connection to spirit and that you are holding great fear in your stomach, probably from an early childhood trauma." She agreed. "There is a cloud of dark energy around your head, probably your constant negative thoughts. Is that accurate?" I asked her. "Yes, that's me," she said, as her mother nodded her head in agreement from the other side of the room.

The palm reading confirmed it. "You have strong healer lines. You are very sensitive: you wear your heart on your sleeve as they say. That makes you an excellent sponge to absorb everybody else's emotions, which you have to be very careful not to take on. You also have strong intuition, as the lines in your moon mountain indicate." "Yes, that's true too. I feel everyone around me," she said. "But, what can I do?" She looked at me confused.

"We will do a cleansing ceremony to remove those negative thoughts and the fear from you, but before that I want to teach you to say no to spirits," I told her. She hesitated. "I don't think I can do that; they are too powerful," she murmured. "They are telling me now not to listen to you and not resist them. I can hear them now; they laugh at me."

"Close your eyes. Can you tell that voice that this is not the right time to communicate with you?" I prompted her. We spent a few long minutes while she struggled to keep her power and authority.

"I also see and talk to spirits freely," I told her. "The only difference between us is that I learned to close those channels of communication when it is not appropriate for me. This is what I will be teaching you to do too." After I performed a cleansing ceremony, she left for home, saying, "I feel lighter, less anxious."

At our next session, her mother left us alone. "There is great improvement in my daughter's behavior and mood. Continue to do what you are doing," she said, before she closed the door behind her.

We started to work deeper on Jennifer's childhood traumas and on her family relationships. She connected with a part of her soul that got confused by her family's constant contradictory expectations of her and the tension in the house. We finished with a cleansing ceremony, to send her home grounded.

For her next session and the ones following, Jennifer decided to take the train to the city by herself, for the first time. "As I was sitting on the train, the voices were trying to discourage me, saying nasty things to keep me from coming to see you. They really don't want me to get better. I closed my eyes and told them to go away. I told them that this is not the right time. It worked. I am here." She was so pleased with her newfound self-confidence.

The last time she came, she was a different person from the one who came to see me a few months before. No longer so shy and was now able to smile freely.

◇ PTSD—Stop Smoking

Paul looked in my eyes with great pride. A big smile spread across his face, as he hugged his big body and gleefully said, "By the way at our last session I forgot to tell you about the two most important things that happened after the session we had before that. First, I finally stopped smoking." His eyes were glowing. "Wow, congratulations!" I exclaimed.

"I think it was those needles you poked me with; it took away all my desire to smoke," he said. "So happy for you," I replied. I gave him a high five across the altar, as it was such a great achievement.

"The other thing was that I felt so much more calm and powerful. It is a new feeling for me. I even sleep better," Paul added, beaming.

When he first came, a few years back, Paul, a Vietnam veteran, was full of rage, hopelessness, anxiety, and paranoia that the world was against him—all signs of PTSD (post-traumatic stress disorder). The Veterans Administration had lost his files and was denying him his benefits. Doctors refused to give him the diagnosis he deserved to get his compensation. He could not find work. His ex-wife had just died, and he felt enormous guilt and responsibility for his two grown-up kids, who themselves had many emotional and physical problems. He blamed his condition and life failure on the Agent Orange he was exposed to in Vietnam.

"I don't want to talk about Vietnam. Don't even ask me," he constantly warned me for months in a metallic tone. "All I want is to have a new wife and maybe start a new family. I want my kids to be able to take care of themselves and build a new life."

It was only after many sessions, using soul retrieval, La Limpia, shamanic journeys, and lots of consultations, which were helpful in getting the Veterans Administration to respond, that he felt comfortable sharing with me some of his traumatic experiences in Vietnam. They were sad stories of great loss—loss of innocence, loss of fellow soldiers, loss of his physical and mental health. But mostly, it was a story of betrayal by his fellow servicemen and commanders. "A cover-up," he said. During many sleepless nights he would mull these betrayals over and over in his head; he couldn't find reasons or make peace with the past.

As he became more optimistic, he brought with him, during separate sessions, his depressed, unemployed, obese son and his troubled daughter who was fighting with her own son over drug use, petty crimes, and missing school. "She has finally take responsibility, and her son has agreed to go to a special program. We'll see. You did what I was not able to do. Thank you," he said after the session with his daughter. It seemed like his life and those of his children had begun to be more balanced.

"Who was that red-haired woman?" I asked him during our last session, reminding him of the candle vision I had had the time before. He giggled. "I've had a fascination with red-haired women since early childhood," he said, red in the face. "I think I may have found one."

◇ Inability to Express Love: It's Never Too Late

It was late afternoon in Warsaw. From the open window of my hotel room, I could see that the sky was turning a dark gray. I was looking forward to relaxing after a full day of sessions. Then the doorbell rang. I was surprised to see Darius, my translator, standing in the doorway. "Yeah, I forgot to tell you that you have one more healing session. This one with a father and son," he said. "But I'm not going to translate. The father prefers that his twenty-five-year-old son, who speaks decent English, translate for him." Soon the two men walked in; the young man was the spitting image of his dad.

"Are you sure that I can ask you intimate questions in the presence of your son?" I asked the father, as we sat down in my small room. He listened to his son's translation of my question, looked deeply at his son, and said, "*Tak, tak.*" Yes, it was okay.

I offered him a white candle. "Let's do a candle reading first," I said. He stood up and rubbed the candle on his body and handed it back to me. In the flame I could see a low-energy man with strong fears concentrated in his stomach. But what was more dangerous was the raging anger he was holding in his body. It seemed that the anger had to do with something that had happened to him at around age six. I now knew what do we needed to work on during the one session I had with him.

"What happened or changed when you were six years old" I asked him. As his son translated, he said, "I started to go to school and my parents left me alone in the house after school. They came late in the evening from their business. They gave me a red string, and on it was a key to wear around my neck." "So who took care of you?" I asked. "No one. Sometimes my grandma came to check on me. I would always justify it by telling myself that they did not have a choice. They had to work to raise me."

"What did you feel?" "I was angry with them and felt abandoned and alone, like nobody cared for me."

"Have you ever been told by your parents that they loved you?" "No," he said with a frozen face and glazed eyes and shook his head. "Did they hug you?" I continued. He took a moment to think, like he was digging deep into his memory bank, hoping to find a treasure. "No. I don't remember. Never." It was so sad to hear that.

"Did you want that?" I asked him. "Yes, of course, but it was not allowed in our house. No one expressed emotions. I never saw them hugging or kissing each other. In our culture it's like that; they assume

that you understand that they love you because they take care of you."
"Did you ever tell this story to your son?" I asked. "No."

"Do you love your son?" I asked him, knowing the son would translate this question for him. "Yes, very much." "Did you ever tell your son that you love him?" His son translated, carefully looking at his father's eyes. "No . . ." He took a deep breath. "I am sorry, son," he said, and he brushed some tears from his eyes. "Would you want to tell him now?" I asked him, as his son translated. "Yes, I think I want to."

There were a few minutes of eerie quietness. "Go ahead, tell him now," I encouraged. The father looked at his son's blue eyes and slowly uttered the three forbidden words: "I love you, my son. I love you so much." He cried as if asking for forgiveness. I looked at the son's face. It was tense and red as he heard those humble words coming from his father's mouth for the first time. My eyes were tearing too.

I decided to push and challenge the father and the son some more. "Would the two of you like to hug?" I asked them. I could see the yearning in the son's body. The father sat there stunned, considering the possibility in his mind. "Go ahead, stand up, face each other, and hug." I encouraged them. I could see there was no turning back.

Slowly, they took a few short steps toward each other. The father first opened his arms and grabbed his son's body firmly. Next the son's arms circled around his father's body. Finally, the two men melted in each other's arms. I could see the trembling in the father's back, as he wept softly, as did his son. I was weeping as well. It seemed like the world was weeping with us, but with joy of the sacredness of that reunion. I felt an awful need to hug my deceased father, who was born not too far from there. It was hard to describe the looks on their faces as they separated and looked at each other. Years of alienation just melted away. They smiled at each other.

"I think we should do a cleansing ceremony now, for both of you," I suggested, and they agreed. So here they were, father and son, being cleansed together. "*Dziękuję* [Thank you]," the father said and gave me a big hug. They left and walked into the cool dark Warsaw night.

A few days later I met them again at my seminar in the Heart &

Mind Festival. They looked so much more at ease with each other and happier together.

A year later I came back to Poland to teach again at the same festival and met them near their shared tent. "How are you doing?" I asked them. They smiled broadly. "We are good. Very good together," the son said. "You know, my father, he is a little crazy." And he chuckled.

◇ *Paranoia and Poison Ivy*

Barbara sat down in a hurry. She lowered her head and played with her long brown hair, then raised her eyes to meet mine. "I don't want you to laugh at me. I am paranoid. It sounds so stupid and trivial, but I can't talk about it with anyone, especially my family. I am so embarrassed even to think of it. I had to see you before it become overblown and ruined my life," she said. "What happened?" I asked her. "Just tell me the facts."

"It sounds so crazy, but every time I walk into my building, the staff treats me with sheer contempt—like, 'Oh, this is that crazy lady again. Be careful of her.' I believe—actually I know—that they installed cameras in my apartment and are watching me. One night the doorman said something to his friend about me that only I could have known. They must have watched me in my apartment."

I've known Barbara for a long time. She is a successful musician and writes musicals and is a great mother for two wonderful boys, so I was utterly surprised to hear her story.

"Instead of talking about it, let's journey and ask your power animal what it's all about," I suggested, and she agreed.

"I had an unusual journey," she said as we sat to discuss it. "My power animal took me to two past lives. It was unexpected. In the first one I was a twelve-year-old girl hiding underground in a sewer during the Holocaust. I could feel the fear and anticipation in my whole body that the German soldiers would find me there. I was in a panic, but I could not express it. I was forbidden to talk.

"In the second lifetime I was a strong muscular man carrying a big, heavy wooden cross on my back. I was walking slowly through a village while a huge crowd heckled me—similar to Jesus, I think."

"I think we now need to do another journey to heal those two life-times," I suggested. "This time I will also journey for you to find the source of that incident." She agreed, and I started to drum.

"My power animal, the horse, ran into a wall and collapsed. A snake or a worm burrowed through the horse and into the earth," she said. "I don't understand that message. Do you? What did you see for me?" She looked into my eyes in confusion.

I told her my vision: "In my journey I saw you as a seven- or eight-year-old girl standing with a group of girls in the schoolyard by a sand-box. I think you were on a break. One of the girls stood up tall on the sandbox ledge and humiliated you in front of all of them from above. I saw you shrinking to a very small, tiny Barbara. The other girls stood there around you quietly in their dresses and said nothing. You were devastated. Does that ring a bell?"

To my surprise she said, "This incident that you just saw was when I was nine years old. I still remember that incident so clearly. That girl you saw was Lesley; she bullied me ruthlessly. I remember that I wanted to shrink and disappear as she made fun of me in front of all my friends. I never could understand why she chose me. Maybe because I was a small girl and so shy and could not protect myself." Her eyes were teary as she continued.

"The funny thing is that a few weeks ago Lesley sent me a friend request on Facebook. I could not believe it. Maybe it brought the whole experience to the surface again. And even more strange was that Lesley's name came up a few days ago in a conversation with my family. We were talking about the dangers of poison ivy, and I told them how a girl named Lesley from my school had told me to rub poison ivy on my face to make myself more beautiful. The next day my face was awfully swol-len and red. Oh, I hated her so much for tricking me. I did not want to go to school, but my mother refused to keep me at home. She sent me to school with that blown-up red face, and it humiliated me to no end. I'm sure Lesley was ecstatic to see me like that," Barbara said angrily.

"OK, now it's time to face Lesley. Let's do a journey," I said.

In the journey, she confronted Lesley and stood her ground. She also had a confrontation with her mother. "I feel I stood my ground. I gained my power back," she said with relief and laughed. "I can't believe that memory brought all this paranoia back into my life. It's so simple."

We finished the session with a cleansing ceremony to remove all that energy from her.

A year or so later Barbara came back. "I'm so distraught; I have to figure it out. Do you think we can do a soul retrieval and see what the problem is?" she asked. We journeyed in tandem. My power animal led me to a house; there, I saw in a darkened kitchen, a young girl around nine years old. Her back was to me. She was peeping through the open door of the dining room, eavesdropping on a group of adults who were sitting around a table set with dishes and food. "This must be her parents and two relatives or friends," I thought. They were conspiring, whispering and laughing maliciously about someone they knew. "Must be a family member they are talking about," I thought, but I could not tell whom. I asked my power animal to find the girl's lost soul part. Immediately I saw her sitting alone on her bed, legs dangling over the side. She was staring in despair through the window at the dark night. "Do you want to come with me and be reinstated with your current Barbara?" I asked her. "I am afraid she will ridicule me too," said the young Barbara. I promised her that Barbara wouldn't, that she actually needed her to feel whole. At last her face changed; she smiled and agreed to come with me. I stopped drumming, held her in the palms of my hands, stood up, and blew her into Barbara's heart and the crown of her head.

"What did you see?" I asked her as we sat facing each other. "I could not journey," she said, apologetically. "But did you see something?" "Yes, something strange," I said and went on to tell her what I had seen. "I'm sorry but I could not understand whom they were talking about." Barbara looked sad and surprised, then took a big breath. I could see her brown eyes getting teary. "I know whom they were talking about. It was about my older cousin, the daughter of my other uncle who was not present at the table. I remember watching them and feeling terrified because they would find out that I am strange and weird too. I was seeing things—remember I told you about the spirits and visions I had as a little girl? My mother did not want to have anything to do with that." "Sure, I remember it very well," I said. "My teenage cousin started taking drugs and alcohol. She dressed odd and became a very strange weirdo. I was afraid they would make me an outcast too. It was frightening. I swore to myself that I would always be a 'good girl' so that no one would gossip about me." She took a deep breath and swept a long brown strand of hair from her face. "Now I understand what that fear was I came to see you about. Wow, thanks for bringing her back."

◇ Frozen with Fear

"You would not believe it. I know it's sound strange, but I have been in three car accidents in the last three years. They all happened the same way: I was a passenger in a car hit in the rear by another car. I am in such a physical mess. I can't understand why it keeps happening to me. Do you think it's a curse?" Suzan looked helpless; a big purplish-blue bruise was still noticeable under her right eye from her last accident.

As it turned out, I discovered, through seeing in the candle flame, that a jealous and vindictive coworker in the adjacent office—a small, dark-haired woman who practiced Santeria—had not only cursed her, but also put magical objects behind her door and between her desk and the wall. (This coworker was later fired, after word of her practices came out in the office.) "Yes, that was true. I found them not long ago." She looked surprised. "I don't know why she did it to me, of all people. I really tried to help her. I bought her lunches and presents for her kids. But I was also afraid of her. I was so afraid to confront her after I found the objects," Suzan said, clasping her hands tightly. "Why did you try to appease her?" I asked her. "I don't really know. It seems like I am helpless, frozen.

"I want to know why am I so frozen, unable to make decisions and afraid of my spiritual side," she said.

"Let's do a soul retrieval," I suggested. "Okay," she agreed. "I have done a few before. Is it possible that one can have many soul parts leave?" "Sure, if a person has had several traumas, it is possible and actually common," I replied.

I began beating the drum; I closed my eyes and called my power animal to take me to a special time when Suzan had experienced a trauma in her childhood. After a few minutes I saw a white cloud hovering in space. It felt very cold. Maybe it was an ice sheet and she was frozen in it, I thought to myself. In the white cloud I saw a little girl about five years old wearing a light dress or a nightgown. She was lying in the middle of the cloud, frozen on her back, her face up and her dark eyes open wide, looking straight up, unable to move her limbs or communicate. That was strange. I could not make out her surroundings or what was the fear all about. I asked my power animal to help me find her lost soul part. It took me out of the window, and there I found a small, beautiful mourning dove on a branch of a tree. I asked the bird if she was Suzan's missing soul part. She confirmed and was very willing to reunite with Suzan. I did not need to convince her: she jumped into my outreached hands. I stopped drumming, hovered over Suzan's body, and blew her spirit into her heart and the crown of her head. We stayed quiet for a few minutes, and I shared my vision with her.

"No, it wasn't ice," Susan corrected me. "When I was about five, like you said, I woke up one night, and there was a white energy cloud above my bed. It had a human face, and I could see piercing eyes looking at me. I was totally terrified. I knew it was not a dream; my eyes were open wide. I could not move; I could not scream. I was literally frozen," she remembered.

"But why a mourning dove?" she wondered. "It is a messenger that connects Mother Earth and Father Sky, or the seen and unseen worlds. It represents true peace and tranquility to a troubled mind affected by trauma and disharmony," I explained. "Oh, I like that," she laughed.

I met Suzan quite often as she embraced her spiritual abilities to heal others and became part of our shamanic community. She did not have any more car accidents in the following years.

◇ Bereavement: Connecting with the Beloved

It was a cruel accident. On his fiftieth birthday this smart and energetic man, a close friend of mine for many years, decided to challenge himself and go deep-water diving with friends. He was a professional diver and was always exceptionally careful. Ed was a smart, unconventional, curious, and joyful man with a big heart and big laugh. But something went awfully wrong, and he died. His family and his friends were in shock.

Many months later, his wife, Lily, came for a healing session. "Do you think I can connect with Ed?" she asked with apprehension. "I feel I never said good-bye. I feel so guilty for letting him go that early morning with his friends. I should not have allowed him. I can imagine his suffering. He left so many projects behind. We worked together, as you know." Lily was seemingly lost in her deep grieving.

The setting was a bit unusual. We were in a hotel room in Florida, as I was teaching that weekend there. So doing a ceremony using traditional methods was out of the question. "Okay, let's try. But first we need to get you a spirit helper, a power animal." I went on to explain what a spirit guide is and how this process works, and she agreed.

Lying on the hotel's big queen-size bed, she covered her eyes and took a big breath. I closed the heavy curtains on the windows from which I could see the blue ocean that took Ed's life and started drumming softly so as not to disturb the hotel guests.

"I think I got it," she said after the drumming stopped. "It was not as hard as I imagined it would be. My power animal, a lioness, says that I need to get stronger, continue on with my life, and most importantly, take care of my two kids. That was awesome." She had a big smile.

"Now, let's try to connect with Ed. You will do another journey, just like the one you did. But now ask your power animal, the lioness, to take you to meet Ed's soul. When you see it, and it can appear in various forms, not necessarily in his image, talk to him, ask him specific questions or advice that only he will know the answers to, and listen to whatever he has to say to you from the other side." And so she did. The drumming went longer this time to give her more time.

"I met Ed. It was so amazing. He appeared much younger, almost the age when we first met years ago. He was smiling and happy," she laughed. "He said not to worry about him, that he is in a good place. He told me he loves me. He told me to continue my work to elect Obama for president. [This was during Obama's election for his first term.] He also told me a few specific things about the computer and our work, which I did not know about; as you know he was the computer geek. That will be very helpful. He said that the accident was not anyone else's fault, which relaxed me, because I suspected it was his partner's fault. Thank you. I think I now have his permission to go on with my life again. I'm so relieved."

Then, gazing at me with her big green eyes, she asked, "But what if I made it all up?" Sitting comfortably on the nice hotel armchair, I smiled and shrugged my shoulders. Finally she took a big breath and answered her own question. "It's not that important. But, that is strange, it does not make sense, how did I get the computer information? I truly have no clue about it. I miss him terribly too."

Epilogue

Taking it from the point of view of Western medicine's scientific logical mind, shamanic healing of course doesn't make much sense. But it works. It produces results that may seem to some of us as if they are incidental miracles. You just can't refute the results. It's not happening by coincidence like many critics claim. I myself am endlessly surprised by it, as are many of my clients as well.

That sentiment is beautifully confirmed by well-known professor Rafi Malach, the Barbara and Morris L. Levinson professorial chair in brain research in the Department of Neurobiology at the Weizmann Institute of Science in Israel, in a personal correspondence regarding our discussions of this book.

It is often stated that brain scientists reduce the depth and beauty of the soul to depressingly simplistic chemical and physical processes—nothing could be further from the truth!

It is precisely because brain scientists relentlessly attempt to better understand the link between the brain and mind that they are repeatedly confronted by how mysterious this link actually is. Indeed, by some alchemy, strictly physical and chemical signals exchange among millions of nerve cells in our brain to magically give rise to our entire inner world with all its richness and vast collections of pictures, memories, emotions, and thoughts. We experience all these so obviously and clearly that it does not cross our minds that behind all these mundane experiences actually lies the deepest mystery facing modern science. The deeper we attempt to understand this process using scientific tools, the more enchanting and miraculous this process reveals itself to be, and the appreciation of this ungraspable phenomenon only deepens our amazement and humility.

So the simple message from neuroscience is that even when in the midst of the most boring moments—say on our way to work or school—it may help to remember that the self-evident picture of a tree or the sky that you happen to look at is in fact a gift given to you by your brain cells in a process that is utterly magical and incomprehensible even to the most knowledgeable brain scientist.

In the journey across the short lifetime we were gifted to be on this Earth, from birth to old age, good physical, emotional, and spiritual health is a crucial, driving force and has been throughout all of our human history. The collective knowledge and wisdom of working with the tangible and spiritual worlds, gathered and treasured by our ancestors, can be an invaluable model for us, and we must be the guardians of this knowledge. As our ancestors did before us, we must recognize and celebrate the deep interconnectedness and codependency of our species with all of nature as the core principle of living life in true happiness and wellness.

As we march into the future, we begin to understand that science and Western medicine with its rapidly developing technologies cannot give us all the answers to the complexities and intricacies of our society and who we truly are. You and I are now part of an amazing conscious revolution that is gaining momentum toward a return to a heart-based society with shared community responsibility.

I strongly believe that only by incorporating shamanic practices and belief systems into a larger vision of well-being can we resolve our emotional and physical problems in the twenty-first century and beyond. I hope you found the information and stories in this book helpful and that you will be able to include them in your daily practice. And please pass them on to your friends, family, and future generations, as our survival depends on it.

Index